Aesthetic Clinic Marketing
in the Digital Age

Aesthetic Clinic Marketing in the Digital Age

Wendy Lewis

President
Wendy Lewis & Co Ltd
Global Aesthetics Consultancy
New York, NY

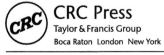

CRC Press
Taylor & Francis Group
Boca Raton London New York

CRC Press is an imprint of the
Taylor & Francis Group, an **informa** business

CRC Press
Taylor & Francis Group
6000 Broken Sound Parkway NW, Suite 300
Boca Raton, FL 33487-2742

© 2018 by Taylor & Francis Group, LLC
CRC Press is an imprint of Taylor & Francis Group, an Informa business

No claim to original U.S. Government works

Printed on acid-free paper

International Standard Book Number-13: 978-1-4987-2672-6 (Paperback)
                                       978-0-8153-6800-7 (Hardback)

Library of Congress Cataloging-in-Publication Data

Names: Lewis, Wendy, 1959- author.
Title: Aesthetic clinic marketing in the digital age / by Wendy Lewis.
Description: Boca Raton, FL : CRC Press/Taylor & Francis Group, [2018] |
Includes bibliographical references and index.
Identifiers: LCCN 2017035457| ISBN 9780815368007 (hardback : alk. paper) |
ISBN 9781498726726 (pbk. : alk. paper) | ISBN 9781498726733 (ebook)
Subjects: | MESH: Cosmetic Techniques--economics | Beauty Culture--economics
| Marketing of Health Services | Social Media--economics
Classification: LCC TT965 | NLM WO 600 | DDC 646.7/2068--dc23
LC record available at https://lccn.loc.gov/2017035457

Visit the Taylor & Francis Web site at
http://www.taylorandfrancis.com

and the CRC Press Web site at
http://www.crcpress.com

Since I began my career in publishing in 2000, this is my twelfth published book penned in my own name (I've ghostwritten more than 20 others for leading physicians), and my first business-to-business (B2B) book written exclusively for healthcare professionals. I am dedicating this book to my brilliant and creative daughter, Eden Lipke, who is my greatest champion. She is my number one sounding board and my "go-to consultant" on all things digital. Her wisdom has been a great asset, keeping me on track and ensuring that my content is fresh and up to date.

Contents

Preface

When it comes to practice marketing, I always enjoy talking to younger physicians because they get it. Their generation grew up online; they are on their mobile devices 24/7 and more than any previous generation; and they understand that digital marketing and media are here and now and will only get bigger in the future.

I offer up best practices for building a website and a blog, pearls on reputation management and how to limit exposure in an open forum, plus share the most relevant social media platforms for aesthetic practitioners, including how to navigate the new social landscape, and they catch on quickly. Whereas, when I address more senior practitioners, it is more of a challenge to get that message across, but that is clearly changing, and they recognize the need to get educated.

Understandably, tweeting, pinning, posting, and blogging can be daunting to any busy aesthetics practitioner. Social media is changing the way patients behave, make purchasing decisions, and see themselves, and also provides a new way for aesthetic practitioners to connect with consumers and to differentiate their clinics. However, to most clinic managers and practitioners, social media represents a sea of confusion that they cannot even begin to know how to navigate. Now with 2 billion monthly users, Facebook remains the biggest social platform globally by a large margin, but it is not the only essential one anymore. Other social platforms of importance to all businesses include Twitter, LinkedIn, YouTube, Instagram, and in some cases, Pinterest and Snapchat. The only constant in the social media world is change.

Marketing is an intensive and challenging activity that requires an understanding of both basic principles and how they can be applied to day-to-day practice. Practitioners need to understand the sweeping changes that are taking place in the market so they don't get left behind. There has been a power shift in the doctor-patient relationship, and the Internet has become the great equalizer. In the digital age, reviews and ratings have the power to persuade or dissuade a patient from choosing one clinic over another. Cosmetic patients are seeking out social networking platforms and online forums to gain information about procedures and to connect with other like-minded individuals to share their experiences and concerns.

This book provides a framework for enhancing the patient experience and understanding marketing segmentation, brand building, innovation, and implementation. Google is not the only game in town; but it is critically important. An integrated social media approach can deliver more return on investment (ROI) than pure search engine marketing alone. It increases community awareness, maintains communication with existing patients, generates referrals, and attracts new patients through word of mouth.

Managing a successful aesthetics clinic requires implementing a marketing plan, developing a cohesive strategy, attracting the right staff with the proper training and expertise, and creating standardized internal processes and techniques.

Offering a high level of patient care and service in addition to effectively marketing your clinic requires a constant, year-round effort. At some point, most practitioners will be faced with deciding between what they are able to do themselves, and what should be outsourced. While aesthetic doctors rarely have time to blog or tweet on a regular basis, social media demands attention 7 days per week, 24 hours per day, and not just when the clinic is open for business. Thus, practitioners need to designate a staff member who has the skill set to manage social media networks and web updates, hire someone to take over the marketing functions in-house, or engage a marketing consultant. Ideally, the practitioner and/or staff can provide the information to the consultant and let the consultant know what is going on in the clinic and how best to promote it. Someone needs to own it.

Despite all the best marketing efforts and expansive programs, many clinics still rely mostly on word of mouth to grow their patient base. In addition, if you ask most practitioners, they will overwhelmingly concur that they get their best patients from referrals from other satisfied patients or colleagues.

But is that really enough to grow your brand sufficiently? Probably not anymore.

If you are not savvy about how to market your clinic online, get educated STAT by attending courses and workshops offered at conferences, network with colleagues, and ask the vendors you deal with for support and assistance. After all, they want you to be successful so you can buy more fillers, lasers, and skin care from them. For larger clinics with multiple practitioners, hiring a marketing manager or clinic director may be the next step to free up time to treat more patients, and increase efficiency and profits.

It is my sincere hope that this book offers some words of wisdom and guidance for you to look at the way you run your clinic in a fresh new way so you can grow.

I look forward to hearing from you, so feel free to reach out. I'm pretty easy to find…

Wendy Lewis
wl@wendylewisco.com
FB wendylewisco
TW wendylewisco
IG wendylewisco

Acknowledgments

I wish to thank the entire team at CRC Press/Taylor & Francis for their tireless patience with me and their undying enthusiasm and support for this book. In particular, I am eternally grateful to Robert Peden, without whose dedication and professional guidance this book would not have been possible. Special thanks must also go to the *PRIME International Journal of Aesthetic and Anti-Ageing Medicine* editorial team, and especially Balraj Juttla.

I must also send a shout-out to my wonderful team of colleagues at Wendy Lewis & Co Ltd, for their endless support, loyalty, and assistance with every project I undertake. And to Denise Mann for being the best editor I have ever worked with.

Disclaimer

The information contained in this book represents the opinions of the author and should by no means be construed as a substitute for legal or financial advice of a qualified professional. The information contained in this book is for general reference and is intended to offer the user general information of interest. The information is not intended to replace or serve as a substitute for any legal or financial professional. Certain content may represent the opinions of Wendy Lewis based on her experience and observations; other consultants may have differing opinions.

All information is provided "as is" and "as available" without warranties of any kind, expressed or implied, including accuracy, timeliness, and completeness. This book is designed to provide information of a general nature about marketing for healthcare professionals, clinics, medical spas, and spas. The information is provided with the understanding that the author and publisher are not engaged in rendering any form of professional services or recommendations. Any information contained herein should not be considered a substitute for professional advice sought for any reader's specific circumstances. Your particular facts, background, circumstances, licensure, scope of practice, and geographic location shall determine the tactics that are most appropriate to your situation. The information contained in this volume is delivered "as is" without any form of warranty expressed or implied. Any use of the information contained within is solely at your own risk. Wendy Lewis & Co Ltd, assumes no liability or responsibility for any claims, actions, or damages resulting from information provided in the context contained herein.

The contents of this book, including but not limited to text, graphics, and icons, are copyrighted property of Wendy Lewis & Co Ltd. Reproduction, redistribution, or modification in any form by any means of the information contained herein for any purpose is strictly prohibited. No part of this book may be reproduced, stored, or introduced into a retrieval system, or transmitted, in any form, or by any means (electronic, mechanical, photocopying, recording, or otherwise), without the prior written permission of both the copyright owner and the publisher of this book.

1

Introduction: Insights on the New Aesthetic Patient Journey

The aim of marketing is to know and understand the customer so well the product or service fits him and sells itself.

Peter Drucker

I started in this field in 1982, and I founded my consultancy in 1997. So, I suppose you can call me a veteran of aesthetic surgery and medicine.

How things have changed since then!

When Marketing Was a Dirty Word

Back when digital marketing was in its infancy, it was unheard of for practitioners of any specialty, cosmetic or otherwise, to have a website or a blog. When Facebook became normalized, it was not considered a primary place to communicate with patients. That came much later. In fairness, the medical profession is not usually the first to jump into new marketing trends. Rather, most practitioners I know take a backseat approach and wait until something goes mainstream to even consider it.

In the evolving digital world, consumers are educating themselves long before they ever get near an aesthetic doctor's clinic waiting room. They often get stuck in a quagmire of information overload and believe they know what they want and need better than the doctor does. They are bombarded with information about medical aesthetic treatments from a wide spectrum of sources, including print, electronic, and broadcast media, websites, physicians, and other specialists.

Cosmetic doctors are not selling a product; they are providing a service—one that is personal and customized to each patient. It is a high-end service that encompasses the entire patient experience. This experience begins with the initial point of contact. In the past, that would have been a telephone inquiry. However, in the digital world, it may be a Google ad, a review on TripAdvisor, or a query on the clinic website. The patient experience then progresses through encounters with the clinic receptionist, assistant, other patients in the waiting room, and the practitioner, thus culminating in a treatment plan, and finally, a treatment.

While the ultimate success of the overall experience is dependent on the practitioner's skill, expertise, bedside manner, and good judgment, there are other factors to consider. Success depends on many tangible and intangible things, including location, accessibility, brand image, the staff, services offered, as well as the culture of the clinic. It is an intensely personal experience.

The High-Tech Clinic

One of the best investments you can make for your practice is to upgrade your technology. Having the right technology in the practice shows patients that you are in the game. Patients do not want to walk into a medical aesthetics clinic to see open files of paper charts strewn around the reception desk. As more physicians are automating routine tasks like recording patient notes, sharing lab results, processing prescriptions, and recording other patient information, technology will play an even more important role in running a clinic efficiently. Offering free Wi-Fi and charging stations for patients, plus monitors, touch screens, and tablets as educational tools is also more common.

The powerful combination of health and technology is changing the way consumers approach their overall well-being. From digital devices that track our every move to online booking engines, digital connectivity is improving the consumer's access to all forms of health and well-being services.

Patients want to have the same kind of efficient experience in your clinic as they have with other businesses. For example, accepting credit and debit cards and Apple Pay is standard in most practices today; also consider using an app so patients can make payments and get their receipts electronically. Offer online bookings, cancellations, and service and product purchasing through your thumb-friendly website and Facebook page. Implement a program to confirm appointments for patient reminders by e-mail or text. Utilize an intake form on an iPad for patients to use while they wait so their information can be entered into your system seamlessly.

These technology hot points are time savers for patients and clinic staff. Technology can also take some of the time-consuming scheduling details out of the experience so patients can sit back and relax. Patients are likely to be most accessible and responsive on their mobile devices. Just keep in mind that if you are going to connect with patients in this way, select an encrypted system that insures that your communications with patients are secure and cannot be intercepted.

The Art of Clinical Photography

Taking good photos before and after procedures is imperative, as patients tend to forget what they looked like before you treated them. If a patient complains that he or she does not see any improvement after her filler or laser, you can whip out the photos and compare them side by side to assess the improvement.

Although we know how difficult it is to get patients to grant permission to share their photos, collecting good clinical photography of your own cases goes a long way to demonstrate the quality of work and results that can be achieved. Many clinics offer tablets in the waiting room or electronic photo frames to display before and after photographs of popular procedures offered in the clinic. This serves as an excellent marketing tool to encourage patients to ask questions about the services you offer. There is no substitute for visuals when it comes to explaining what having two syringes of a hyaluronic acid filler may look like on the patient's cheeks, or how much visible improvement can be achieved after a series of nonablative fractionated laser treatments.

Reviews and Your Reputation

Like it or loathe it, consumers have become programmed to check reviews before they go, buy, or choose when it comes to products and services. Negative content posted about healthcare practitioners can directly affect the success of their practices, as more consumers rely on ratings and reviews to select their doctors, and to rule out the ones they don't want to go to. In the digital world, consumers are inclined to speak their minds and share their opinions about your practice, whether they are fair or not. Historically unhappy patients tend to be the most vocal, which makes the system that much more frustrating.

Doctors have always been the beneficiaries and victims of ratings; they just were not online and in our faces. They have always had positive and negative comments, but the forum has expanded from bridge clubs and locker rooms to the online universe.

Social media has proven to be a great outlet for physicians to help educate consumers, showcase innovative procedures, and demonstrate their expertise. But I would strongly encourage you to play it safe. All licensed healthcare professionals should establish their own professional profiles and keep their personal activities online off limits for patients. This tactic will assist in controlling the amount of accurate information that is out there for patients to discover online and help to maintain your reputation as a professional.

The stakes are higher now due to increased competition, and every patient counts. Aesthetic practitioners need to market themselves, which makes them more vulnerable to these kinds of attacks from all sources. Ignore them at your own peril.

Delivering Five-Star Service

Clinics that provide a great experience tend to be rewarded over the long term by customer loyalty. Those that don't are shooting themselves in the proverbial foot.

Over time, there is long-term value in delivering a great experience, and it is rewarded by consumers who send their friends and family to your clinic and tell people about you. Poor customer service hurts the clinic's overall performance, drives down revenue, increases costs, and undermines staff morale, which causes turnover. In short, customer frustration leads to more employee attrition and higher operating expenses.

If you look at customer service as just another expense in your budget rather than an investment, you will be more inclined to cut back during slow periods to improve the bottom line. This strategy will work against you in the long term. We know that it costs much more to attract new patients than to maintain the ones you already have. If good service is an afterthought at your clinic, you are making a huge mistake. In an era when the same products and services are offered by so many competing clinics, a key point of differentiation rests on how you treat patients and on good customer service. People are more likely to remember a negative experience, and they are also more willing to talk about it to their friends and broadcast it online.

It costs much more to bury negative reviews than to generate positive ones. This does not factor in the angst of dealing with unhappy, vocal patients. Providing customers with a meaningful, memorable, and enjoyable experience is the gift that keeps on giving. Clinics should also understand the link between the patient and the staff. A central part of every clinic should include an emphasis on staff training to make sure that everyone is up to speed on every service, procedure, and product offered, and feels like they are working toward a common goal. When your staff loves what they do and like each other, they are in a better position to make patients feel welcome and happy to be there. This, in turn, creates more engaged staff, patients, and referrals.

Sometimes it costs more up front to do the little things that benefit your patients—such as providing a favorable pricing strategy, offering liberal scheduling, adding more staff, or upgrading your clinic waiting room—but the rewards come on the back end. Rethink the way you run your clinic. You can never go wrong by taking great care of your patients. That strategy will always pay you back for years to come. But when you look at turnover and training costs and customer satisfaction, there are also a lot of advantages to having happy, enthusiastic, and loyal employees, and paying them well is one of the things that helps keep them happy.

Consider the 80/20 rule: 20% of patients generate 80% of your revenue.

If your clinic impresses your patients, you will benefit by gaining loyal patients who become your advocates. Patients will also spend more with you and be more open to sharing their positive experience with others.

2

Fundamentals of Clinic Marketing

Great things in business are never done by one person. They're done by a team of people.

Steve Jobs

A marketing program should be based on looking at your clinic in terms of your patients' needs and their satisfaction; whereas selling is all about techniques to get people to buy your product or service. The inherent difference is that marketing is an integrated effort that is in line with your core business model. To maintain visibility, aesthetic clinics should have a consistent presence across a variety of channels that are relevant to the segment of patients they want to reach. In essence, your clinic needs to be visible where your patients are. Just having a clinic website and a Facebook page is not sufficient. These are only two spokes of the grand marketing wheel.

A strong marketing plan will increase your clinic's visibility and profile, maintain communication with patients, and encourage referrals of new patients due to the high quality of care you deliver. Before investing in getting new patients in the door, determine if you have the right staff, if you have enough staff, if staff members need some additional training, if your location is convenient and nice enough for your target audience, and if you have the right menu of services to meet their needs. You also need to figure out what needs to be added or changed to allow you to expand your reach.

MUST-HAVE MARKETING TOOLS

1. Updated and optimized website
2. Mobile website
3. Pay-Per-Click advertising
4. Public relations campaign
5. Facebook page
6. Blog
7. Twitter
8. Instagram
9. Open House events
10. Community outreach
11. Monthly specials
12. E-mail marketing
13. Patient rewards program
14. YouTube channel
15. LinkedIn listing

THE 5 P'S OF CLINIC MARKETING

Positioning—Choosing the best positioning for your clinic to reach your target audiences

- Is your clinic high volume/low price, low volume/high price, or middle of the road?

- How is your practice differentiated from your competitors?
- Are you ready to change your positioning?

People—Building a clinic team of rock stars

- What do your patients expect from the services you offer?
- Is your clinic team meeting or exceeding those expectations now?
- Do you need to expand, change, or retrain your team?

Price—Setting your value proposition and fee structure

- How do you calculate the value of the products and services you offer?
- Are there established price ranges in your local area?
- Do your competitors offer discounts, special packages, or bundle products and services?
- How does your pricing strategy compare to your top competitors?

Products—Reevaluating your menu of products and services

- What does your brand currently offer?
- What is missing from your menu of services to address any unmet needs?
- What products or services are patients asking for most?
- What will complement your menu to increase average sales and profits?

Promotion—Developing and implementing a marketing plan and budget

- Digital marketing, social media
- E-mail marketing, patient seminars
- Public relations
- How do your competitors promote their clinics?

Consumers are educating themselves, so you need to make it easy for patients to find you online. This is called *inbound marketing*, which is defined simply as the process of helping potential patients find your clinic before they are ready to make a purchasing decision, and then leveraging that early awareness of your clinic to stay in their minds for when they are ready to make a purchasing decision (i.e., book a consultation, schedule a treatment, or purchase a product).

Branding Your Clinic

A brand and its ability to influence consumer behavior are based on the customer experience, rather than solely on the marketing and promotional activities behind it.

Studying the behavior of big brands can be misleading largely because the rules under which they operate are simply not applicable to an average aesthetic clinic. Do you have a marketing and design department? Do you have a budget with multiple zeros? Do you have in-house information technology (IT) expertise? Do you have the ability to hire multiple vendors to make your marketing sizzle? Global powerhouses like Apple, Nike, and Coca-Cola tend to be public companies with vast corporate structures and big budgets.

If your clinic offers the same treatments and services as every other clinic, you cannot really compete on the basis of branding alone. To differentiate your clinic, offer something that not everyone else can offer—a unique product or personalized service. It is about the people, not just the products. People cannot be duplicated.

Customer loyalty and a growing customer base will not emerge from branding exercises alone. They have to evolve from the quality of the care provided and the total customer experience. This does not mean that you do not need a memorable name, attractive logo and color scheme, and modern clinic design and flow. These are also keys to success in the business of aesthetic medicine.

Defining Your Clinic Brand

A brand for a company is like a reputation for a person. You earn reputation by trying to do hard things well.

Jeff Bezos

Your brand determines your competitive advantage, and it is a vital asset that should be protected at all costs. It exemplifies your reputation among patients, colleagues, and influencers. By building brand equity, you can distinguish your aesthetics clinic from all the others in the market that offer similar services. Branding is about more than just putting up a sign, creating a logo, or the facility and location. It is about who you are as a practitioner, the reputation you have earned among your patients, your core competencies, and the service culture your clinic offers.

Your value proposition or unique selling point is what sets your clinic apart from the clinic across the road or the chain of clinics springing up within your zip code. This encompasses your strengths and unique training, high quality of care, specialization in a particular treatment category, convenience and comfort of location, or a one-stop shopping experience. Your unique selling point is a combination of factors that you can point to as making your clinic better or at least different than all of the others. It is that point of differentiation that will enable you to rise above your competition.

Sophisticated consumers tend to seek providers with a difference that resonates in terms of value, prestige, and service. Establish a fundamental platform of key messages about what you do differently or better and what makes your clinic ideally suited for your target audience's needs. Survey what your competitors are doing, and determine what you offer that is superior. Always aim to up your game to stand out.

Your brand depends on what comes to mind when patients think about your clinic as a result of the total impressions made by encounters with your brand name, logo, website, marketing, advertisements, and everything else that people see and hear about your clinic. Even basic things like the clinic entrance and curb appeal contribute to how your brand is perceived. Every time someone walks past your clinic, sees your Google ad, encounters a staff member, or reads about you, he or she is forming a lasting impression about your brand.

Looking at your clinic through patients' eyes will help you define your brand. Align everything you offer with what your clinic actually delivers. If this does not line up, there is a gap that needs immediate attention. For example, if you are promoting a body-shaping treatment that you are calling, "Lunchtime Lipo," and the patient winces in pain and leaves with such severe bruising that she cannot go back to work for a few days, the trust factor for your clinic brand will suffer.

Setting a Fee Structure

A key component of branding is to determine your positioning in the marketplace. Decide if you want your clinic to be high volume and low cost, or low volume and premium pricing. The former requires a fairly substantial expenditure on marketing to keep a steady stream of new patients coming in, whereas the latter may be best accomplished by investing in public relations activities and forming referral relationships with like-minded practitioners of other specialties. The safe zone is to be somewhere in the middle—average volume and average pricing.

WENDYISM

Price is just a dollar amount, but value is the relative worth or desirability of a product or service to the end user.

Competing on price is always a losing proposition; there will always be someone who is willing to offer the same or similar service or product for a lower profit. Find out what other clinics are charging in your local community for the same or similar treatments. Try to establish a belief among your patients that they are receiving good value from your practice. Instead of cutting prices and thereby reducing profits, offer more in terms of services, convenience, aftercare, and pampering.

Whatever route you take, stay true to your brand.

THE GROUPON TRAP

Consider this scenario. You find out from one of your patients that the practice down the block sent out an e-blast offering 40% off every laser treatment for the month of November. You go into panic mode and start slashing your fees to compete, offering 50% off every laser treatment. You call your webmaster to post this special offer on your website, send out an e-blast, and post it on your Facebook page.

What is wrong with this picture? You have fallen into the Groupon trap and it is not pretty. By taking this approach, you are being reactive rather than proactive. In essence, you are responding to what your competition is doing instead of setting the standard yourself. Rather than beating your competition, you are basically adopting the same strategy. The cost of this exercise may outweigh any possible benefits. You may be discounting your fees so much in addition to outspending your competition, that your campaign will be too successful—you may end up doing more treatments but losing money on every treatment!

Furthermore, you have unwittingly set a new precedent. By reducing fees on your services, you have essentially devalued your time and expertise, and patients may come to expect more deep discounts in the future. In fact, those patients are being trained to just wait for the next time you have a panic attack and slash your prices.

By adapting the same marketing tactics that your competitors are using, you are missing a prime opportunity to differentiate yourself in the market. The knock-on effect is that you are in danger of commoditizing your services. We know that one laser treatment does not equal another. The exact point of difference may lie in the quality of the technology, the expertise of the practitioner, and the results that are achieved. Another point of difference is the level of service, care, comfort, and convenience offered. Rather than cutting your fees to match your competitors, elevate your brand so customers understand why you are better and worth the higher fees.

Reconsider the same scenario. You find out that the practice down the road sent out an e-blast offering 40% off every laser treatment for the entire month of November. You plan your strategy based on facts instead of raw fear, ego, or emotion. You find out what lasers your competitor has and delve deeper into the specific details of this offer. You may actually learn that it is 40% off a series of six laser hair removal treatments, which amounts to the same price as the usual fee of six laser hair removal treatments for the price of five, and that it is only offered on Friday afternoons between 3 and 5 PM. You then craft an e-blast to your patients, and post on your Facebook page that your practice is launching a new state-of-the-art laser treatment that addresses a common concern such as diffuse redness or sun damage to cast a wide net. This treatment can be positioned as your loss leader—that is, a relatively inexpensive treatment on which your profit margin is low that is offered to attract new customers into your practice.

This offers a fresh core message with a unique point of differentiation—new technology that is faster or more precise, effective treatments that address common issues among patients interested in laser procedures, and a good value proposition. Rather than running with the default message of lower prices, offering good value is a superior path that will not cheapen your brand.

Value is subjective; good value to one customer may not be the same as good value to the next. Once these core messages have been tailored to match your short-term as well as long-term goals, they should be communicated throughout an integrated marketing campaign.

Internal Marketing

By definition, *internal marketing* involves promoting your services to the internal customers of the practice. This concept has evolved to include communications to existing customers, or patients, who already know your practice. Internal marketing can be facilitated in many ways and should be a consistent theme to keep your practice on your customers' minds and instill patient loyalty.

Word of Mouth

Word of mouth is still the most effective way to market your clinic. The act of consumers talking to other consumers about your clinic generates exposure for your brand among prospective patients who may not otherwise know of you. But for word-of-mouth marketing to be effective, you have to give patients good reason to talk about your products and services. It is the art and science of building active, mutually beneficial consumer-to-consumer and consumer-to-clinic communications.

It is well accepted that word of mouth is the most trusted form of marketing because the person providing the recommendation has used the service or product and is speaking from personal experience. Generating positive word of mouth for your clinic is a constant challenge, especially when patients are not always inclined to broadcast the fact that they have received aesthetic treatments. Happy, satisfied customers are less likely to go public or write glowing reviews and endorsements, whereas disgruntled patients tend to be more vocal, proactive, and demanding.

Enabling recommendations, referrals, reviews, and testimonials from patients by delivering good service and superior outcomes should be a continuous process. In a crowded market, you need to work even harder to keep patients happy, meet or exceed their expectations, and deliver consistent results. This involves listening to your patients, engaging them in a dialogue through multiple platforms, and empowering them to tell their friends and family about you.

This sharing of information may take place online in forums, blogs, and review sites, as well as in the form of personal letters, testimonials, and daily conversation. Harnessing the power of advocates to promote your brand can expand your reach organically.

The flipside is that managing a dissatisfied customer is just as important so they are *not* vocal which can severely tarnish your brand's reputation. Dealing with vocal critics and chronic complainers is a critical issue for all practitioners, especially since negative reviews can leave an indelible black mark on your standing among prospective patients.

Identify loyal customers who may agree to be your advocates to carry your key messages to others. Building brand visibility by turning patients or customers into advocates is a main driver for launching a comprehensive social media marketing program. Your brand advocates on Facebook, Twitter, and other social media platforms can help you get the word out and can increase the return on investment (ROI) of your social media efforts. With the rise of social media, the speed and reach of word-of-mouth communications has increased significantly.

This outreach should be sincere and transparent. It must come from the hearts of customers and patients who are genuine cheerleaders for your practice because they truly believe in you. Do not attempt to fake it; this can backfire badly. It is manipulative and deceitful, and consumers are much too smart to be fooled so easily.

Customer satisfaction drives referrals, and these referrals must be handled well to generate more referrals. Never take loyal customers for granted, but rather continue to strive to earn and maintain their confidence in your practice.

E-mail Marketing

The reports of the death of e-mail marketing are greatly exaggerated.

E-mail is not yet dead, but rather it needs to be smarter and stronger than ever to deliver the right content to the right people at the right time. E-mail marketing continues to be one of the top performing tactics in your marketing toolbox. You can use data to improve the quality of your e-mail lists, and e-mail marketing and automation make up a dominant powerhouse driving consistent, engaging, revenue-producing campaigns that can be accomplished in house.

If you are not using e-mail marketing, you are missing out on one of the best ways to reach patients who know you. For sharing news, highlighting products and services, and enticing consumers with promotions, e-mail marketing campaigns are cost effective and easy to create, and they offer plenty of opportunities to measure success.

One form of internal marketing that is a mainstay is distributing newsletters by e-mail to past and present patients. This is a well-accepted method of keeping in contact with patients. To set this program in motion, you need an up-to-date e-mail database that patients have opted into. E-blasts can include newsworthy and timely articles, monthly specials, and tidbits of clinic news. The goal is to stay relevant and visible to your patients as their preferred aesthetics provider when they are ready to have a treatment.

E-blasts are best timed at specific intervals, but not so often as to cause the recipients to mark them as spam or opt out of your mailing list. Monthly is a safe model to follow. Many clinics also use printed newsletters that are handed out in the clinic, supplied to referral partners, and/or mailed out on a quarterly basis. Clearly, print runs are more expensive, but they can have a longer shelf life.

Affordable e-mail marketing solutions that you can take advantage of are readily available. These services enable you to see exactly who is opening your e-mails, and who is actually reading what was sent. As with other forms of marketing, clinic owners can use e-mail marketing to build brand loyalty, find new customers, and encourage repeat business.

HOW TO USE E-MAIL MARKETING

- **E-blasts or newsletters:** A quick way to keep your current patients informed of any clinic news or upcoming promotions. Newsletters should be sent on a recurring basis, such as monthly or quarterly.
- **Promotional campaigns:** Used to let customers know about upcoming offers, new services, and products. They can be sent in the days or weeks leading up to the date to keep patients in the loop.
- **Invitations:** Keep patients informed of special events. Invitation e-mails can be sent weeks before an event as a way to encourage RSVPs and add "Bring a Friend" with a link to share or forward to spread the word.
- **Lead generation:** Designed to keep your brand foremost in the minds of prospective patients and can be sent on a regular basis to encourage treatment trial and conversion.
- **Surveys:** Prepare short e-mail surveys as a way to learn more about your patients' needs and wants. These may also be used as patient satisfaction surveys to determine how you are doing in the eyes of your patients.

- **Transactional e-mails:** Sent after a purchase is made either online or in the clinic, as a way to confirm the transaction and thank the patient for his or her business.

Among the advantages of e-mail marketing over other strategies is cost, which is a key differentiator. E-blasts can be sent for free or at a low cost. They can be designed and sent in a few days in house, as opposed to taking weeks to plan and execute. Most platforms also provide greater tracking tools and analytics.

There are many services and programs designed to help create professional campaigns and track results so that you can gauge the effectiveness of your messaging. You will be able to see which e-mails were received, which went to addresses that were no longer active, which were actually opened, which were deleted before they were read, and which enticed clients to click through to the website. The main drawback to e-mail marketing is that many recipients can consider the e-mails to be spam and opt out of receiving more. If they feel as though they are being bombarded by unwanted e-mails, they will be less likely to become a new or repeat customer. They may also report you to the e-mail service, which can present major hurdles.

Before you send e-mail blasts, you must get patients' permission to do so.

ANTI-SPAM LAWS

Anti-spam laws regulate spamming tightly, and if you violate these policies, you will be at risk of getting banned from the e-mail service you are using. To avoid these problems, build a solid e-mail list, and make sure that patients have signed up to receive your e-blasts. Many companies now use a double opt-in process that requires users to click a confirmation link on an e-mail generated after they have signed up.

Make sure to comply with the rules and regulations in effect where you practice.

E-mail marketing services may provide the software and tools needed to create and execute e-mail marketing campaigns. Specifically, they feature templates to use to design and create all types of e-mail marketing campaigns. The design tools are created so that even those who do not have graphic design experience can easily develop something eye catching and professional. They also help to collect and store e-mail addresses and that keep track of what happens with each e-mail sent. The data and statistics simplify your ability to determine the success of a campaign.

Fees vary by provider, and pricing plans are usually based on the number of e-mails that will be sent out each month. Choose a service that offers an extensive feature list, including user-friendly campaign wizards and templates, options that show what an e-mail will look like, and the ability to test certain word choices to avoid getting flagged as spam. The best services offer robust campaign reporting options that provide everything from click-throughs, conversions, replies, forwards, opened e-mails, bounced e-mails and subscribed/unsubscribed numbers, and online or phone support.

8 GREAT E-MAIL MARKETING PLATFORMS

- Campaignmonitor.com
- Constantcontact.com
- Getresponse.com
- Icontact.com
- Klaviyo.com
- Mailchimp.com
- Paperlesspost.com
- Verticalresponse.com

Even in the era of social media, virtually everyone who is online still has at least one e-mail address, usually one for business and another for personal mail. Most of us check our accounts at least a few times a day for new messages, and it is still the primary way people communicate in business, at least for now. But tech-savvy consumers have grown wise to the typical tactics that fill their inboxes with ads and promotions. To catch their attention, you have to go above and beyond.

E-mail blasts are an ideal way to spread your brand's message to loyal patients who already want to hear from you. Provide a quick and convenient way to subscribe to your e-mail messages with a strategically placed sign-up form on your site's landing page.

Align your brand's message with a beautiful design with the help of e-mail marketing services that offer professionally designed templates. These tools allow you to easily add images, tweak margins, and edit the template colors to match your brand.

You need to stay on top of your e-mail list to keep it current. Many services offer a suite of tools to help you manage and grow your lists to connect with current patients who have opted in and reach new ones. They also help you to avoid sending duplicate e-mails and automatically remove unsubscribes. They can help grow your lists by capturing new contact information from your website, Facebook or Instagram, and other sites.

It is a good idea to tailor your messages to different audiences. For example, you can pitch one message to patients who have not been in for a year or more, and another message to active patients, or segment your database in another way. Your carefully crafted e-mail campaign can fall apart if your messages go to the wrong people at the wrong times. Utilize automation tools that can help get your plan executed. Create a custom calendar to send time-based messages at optimum days and times. Subscribers can receive your e-mails on the weekend, birthdays, or anniversaries.

With analytics tools, you can track subscriber responses and give unsuccessful strategies the boot. Automatically generated reports will help you decide which e-mail messages give your business the best ROI. That information can help you tailor messages and promotions to maximize engagement with potential customers. Some services make it easy to share a promotion on Facebook, Twitter, or LinkedIn with a single click, or to create your own coupons for selected patient groups to help you target future promotions more effectively.

Calls to Action

Calls to action (CTAs) are one of the key lead generation elements of both traditional and digital marketing. In a perfect world, all or most of your marketing tactics (social media updates, press releases, blog posts, e-blasts, newsletters, invitations, etc.) should include some form of CTA.

A CTA should be designed to appeal to your target audience so that they take the action you want them to take. For example, it should compel the reader to do something, such as click, call, or schedule. Your website should have a CTA also, in the form of a response you want users to complete. This may include filling in a contact form, signing up for a newsletter, or downloading an e-book. The CTA should be placed where it will get noticed and include words that encourage users to take definitive action.

To take your CTA one step further, create a sense of urgency by adding phrases to encourage the user to act immediately. Another way to create a sense of urgency is to offer extra benefits to those who sign up early, or refer their friends and family.

ACTIVE WORDS AND PHRASES

Shop	Call
Register	Share
Sign up	Offer expires by (Add date here)
RSVP	For a limited time only
Subscribe	Order now to receive a free gift
Click	Space is limited

View	Valid for 30 days
Enter to win	Introductory offer
Schedule	The first 10 people who respond…

Positioning Your Call to Action

The position of the CTA on your landing page, e-blast, or ad is equally important. Ideally, it should be placed high on the page and in the central column to be readily seen. The more space around a CTA, the more attention may be drawn to it. If your CTA is located where there are too many other features to distract the user, it may get lost. The position, color, and white space surrounding your CTA are all keys to success.

The bigger your CTA, the more chance it will be noticed. A CTA should not just be limited to the home page. Every page of your site should have some form of CTA that leads the user on. Your CTA does not need to be the same for each page. Instead, you can use smaller actions that lead the user toward your ultimate goal.

> If you require users to provide personal data, avoid asking for information that is not a "must have" but a "want to have." Although there is value in data, there is a high probability that users will drop out of the process without completing it, so it may not be worth the risk. Keep the "nice to have" fields optional and only basic information mandatory.

Before someone may complete a CTA, he or she has to recognize the benefits of responding. Think about what the user will get out of it and how you are going to communicate that benefit. You need to clearly explain what the user will gain by taking the desired action. In some cases, you may add incentives to encourage users to complete a CTA. These may include discounts, entry into a competition, or a free gift.

Keep it simple. If you have too many CTAs, patients may become overwhelmed and opt out. A customer who is presented with too many options is less likely to pursue your CTA or make a purchase. By limiting the number of choices, you avoid confusion and make it simpler for users to take advantage of the offer. Monitor how many clicks it takes to act on the offer, and consider how to streamline the process.

An effective CTA can generate measurable ROI. Think about what happens when a user responds to your CTA. The rest of the process should be carefully designed so the back end is seamless, and the promised benefits are provided in a timely fashion. Make sure your e-mail blasts are in line with the overall tone and messaging of your brand for consistency.

Measuring Success

To judge how well an e-mail campaign works, look at how many people opened it, forwarded it, clicked through to your website, and actually converted. Check your analytics to see if you are getting better open rates with each e-blast sent. You cannot expect a high conversion just from one e-mail; it will take a few to gain momentum. Aim for a high interaction rate from current patients, and as your list grows, more people will be interested to go to your website and consider having a consultation or treatment.

Craft a strategy for a year by determining what you want to send and what each e-blast will promote. Select your target audience, consider how you will get their e-mails, and segment them. Then contemplate your goals for the campaign and integrate it with all your other marketing efforts. Start by focusing on your core client base rather than chasing new clients. The return has much bigger potential.

A series of ads running at consistent intervals is always more effective at building brand identity than one random ad, and the same principles apply here.

Do not spam your list. When someone signs up to receive a newsletter, send out one confirmation e-mail to welcome that person. Try not to start bombarding subscribers with a constant stream of sales pitches and aggressive messages—that tactic is so 2007. It will come across as desperate and offensive, which results in nasty responses like "Take me off your list!" or unsubscribes.

The next frontier emerging is text messaging, Facebook messaging, WhatsApp, and other messaging platforms that are definitely on the rise for businesses wishing to connect with customers.

Open House Events

Open house events are a mainstay among successful aesthetic clinics. Typically, this strategy is more effective in smaller cities and suburban areas, where there are fewer distractions than in major cities like New York or London. Clinic events can range from small and intimate gatherings of people who are very motivated to have a treatment to large groups who have brought along their friends.

Educational seminars and events are a great way for established patients to learn about different cosmetic procedures and products your clinic offers. Evening hours are the most popular time to host events, and Tuesdays, Wednesdays, and Thursdays tend to work best. You can serve a signature cocktail, or wine and snacks, or go with coffee or tea and sweets. Some clinics do live demonstrations so patients can check out different procedures and learn how they work. Guests have the opportunity to ask patients questions about the procedure, pain level, what it feels like, and see photos of actual patients' results.

Open house seminars should be developed around seasonal or timely themes, such as "Brighten Up Your Skin for Spring," or "Shape Up for the Holidays." In some cases, representatives from vendors may be invited to support the event. A brief slide presentation is helpful for guests to learn more about what the clinic offers. Patients should be encouraged to schedule a consultation for more information, and take home goody bags with samples and brochures.

Patient seminars raise awareness and can generate appointments. These events attract not only potential patients, but also those interested in other treatment options (a halo effect), which can make a significant impact on clinic growth. They also help to position your clinic as a leader in medical aesthetics within the community.

Successful seminar programs require careful planning, flawless logistics, and brilliant execution from the pre-event planning phase to post-event follow-up.

Getting the Word Out

Start promoting your event at least 3 weeks, preferably 6 weeks, in advance with a "save the date" notice. Add seminar program details on your website, Facebook business page, Instagram, and Twitter feed. Submit event details to local online news sites and event calendars for posting to the local community.

Suggested targets may include women over 50 interested in antiaging treatments, "soccer moms" concerned with post-baby body shaping, or professional women looking for discreet maintenance. In my experience, it is harder to get men to come to patient seminars. Seminar topics should specifically feature the benefits of what your clinic offers in a few key areas. Promoting broader topics is not always as effective in generating interest and attendance. For example, use events to introduce new treatments and technologies, or a group of treatments that work well together, such as toxins and fillers or lasers and peels. Don't go too broad with your theme and throw too many topics and offers at attendees. Keep it focused.

Venues should be accessible and offer convenient parking or access to public transport. Events are best held within your clinic, space permitting. This helps keep costs down and allows for a more personalized and intimate atmosphere.

Before the Event

Establish scripts for RSVP calls that ask how consumers learned about your event and your clinic. This provides valuable information on marketing effectiveness and will allow you to tailor future events to maximize ROI. Seminar advertisements with targeted messages are essential to successful events. For example, messages that emphasize key catchphrases, such as "Learn how to take 10 years off your face (no surgery required)," to highlight injectables, a laser and skincare solution, can boost attendance and leads than messages that are less enticing or too vague.

At the Event

Several strategies can be used to capture appointments, depending on the regulations in the area where you practice and the clinic guidelines. Assign a staff member to check in all guests upon arrival and book appointments on request. "Thank you for attending" follow-up e-mails should be sent after the event to encourage guests to schedule. In many markets, a special offer is promoted at the event to encourage a trial. Patients may be invited to take advantage of a limited time offer—such as 20% off a treatment or product selection—that must be paid for at the event for services to be used within a specific period, such as 30–90 days after the event.

Live Patient Demo or Video

Invite happy patients to speak with attendees about their procedures, the results, and the impact the procedures have had on their lives. Connecting guests with real patients can greatly influence the decision-making process. Doing a demo or playing a video of satisfied patients before the seminar starts is a great attention-grabbing strategy to spark early interest in the procedures you are promoting. It is also good to invite local media to introduce them to your clinic.

After the Event

Seminars attract interested prospective patients, which can directly office visits. Attendees should be tracked to examine how many make office appointments and the procedures performed to judge ROI. Conducting seminars and events that introduce new patients to your clinic maximizes lead generation and drives procedure and sales uptick. Conversion rates will depend on multiple factors, including planning, location, theme, time of year, and so on. Using proven marketing strategies to generate buzz improves attendance and enhances the outcome.

PATIENT SEMINAR PROMOTION

- Multiple seminar marketing promoting a series of one to four seminars on different topics
- Serial e-mail blasts spaced at least 1 week apart
- Integrated Facebook/Instagram event promotion—boosted posts, sponsored content, invitation, Facebook event posting on business page
- Blog before and after the event with images (excluding patient photos)
- Feature a "What's New" section on the website or landing page
- Invitations provided to local partners or affiliates for their customers (salons, spas, gyms, etc.)
- Listings on local event calendars online
- Banner ads on local news sites, community bulletin boards

External Marketing

The days when you could just hang up a shingle and develop a successful practice are long gone. Practitioners must also be strong marketers to succeed, no matter how good they are in the technical aspects of their profession.

Many practitioners get discouraged from past experiences of tactics that have not produced results. They may have tried something once or twice that did not meet their expectations and then abandoned the strategy. It is well known that marketing is not a one-shot deal. It should be consistent and be part of an integrated strategic plan.

Instead of hard core traditional advertising, think of your marketing as consumer messages that are positioned in the more relaxed style of a conversation between friends, or branded or sponsored content. These strategies can help build and maintain long-term relationships with patients. Your overriding goal should be to get patients to like and trust you. If you succeed, they will remember you when they, or any of their circle of family and friends, need what you offer.

Many clinics invest heavily in paid online advertising options to generate leads. Your competitors may already be advertising and capturing market share at your expense. If none of your competitors are advertising online yet, that may be the most compelling reason for you to start. Strike a delicate balance between tasteful, professional campaigns that maintain your integrity and positioning as a physician. In many markets, the governing bodies have cracked down on programs designed to aggressively lure patients into aesthetic clinics.

Integrated marketing draws on the power of traditional methods, such as web marketing, advertising, and public relations, and merges them with search engine optimization, Pay-Per-Click ads, and social media. Integrating your marketing programs involves creating a central theme and imagery that defines your brand and is cohesive. For example, the look and feel of your blog should complement your Facebook page and the landing page of your website. Websites and blogs should have links to every other platform the practice is engaged on, including Facebook, Twitter, LinkedIn, YouTube, and Instagram. All content can be shared, adapted, and recycled across every other platform you participate in for maximum exposure. The key is to avoid duplicating content because that can work against you with search engines.

So, You Want to Be a Media Darling

Public relations (PR) is a brand awareness booster.

Although you cannot always measure the precise ROI from PR exposure, patients will remember that they saw you quoted in a magazine or on a talk show. This heightens your credibility and may be the deciding factor for a patient who has heard about you in persuading him or her to schedule a visit. If you have TV or print coverage on a specific procedure, that may give your clinic a big boost in new patients.

A good PR firm with experience and current contacts in the health and beauty media, can give you access to editors, producers, bloggers, and journalists who have the clout to enhance your brand. You can try to manage media outreach in your local market in house, but success will be limited. For example, sending out press releases on newswires when you have something of interest to broadcast, such as a new technology or clinical study.

Newspapers and online magazines have a constant need for fresh content. Your staff may be able to pitch you as a skin expert, or to write a column or feature articles on timely skin tips or sun protection, acne, and more. National television segments have stiff competition; however, there may be opportunities in your local market. A 5-minute spot on your local news can be very compelling to patients who already know you, and it serves as a reinforcement of your leadership in the field. It can also drive new patients who are intrigued by what they heard, read or saw into your clinic.

Traditional media functions are to inform, persuade, entertain, investigate, educate, and earn a profit. To be successful at telling your story, your relationship with the media should be symbiotic—that is, mutually dependent and mutually beneficial. They want news, and you want to be part of that news. If your news is interesting, accurate, and dependable over time, you are on the right track.

Research into and knowledge of the topic presented in a clear, concise, and honest manner will help you gain trust and credibility in the future. Present your information accurately while adding a creative twist that will appeal to the audience. Get to know publishers, editors, reporters, and bloggers. Your role is to inform, attract, and gain support from them. Their role is to attract the reader or listener.

10 TIPS FOR WORKING WITH THE MEDIA

- Understand their deadlines and respond as soon as possible.
- Respect their busy schedule by asking, "Is this a good time for you?" or "Can we schedule a time to talk?"
- Learn how they like to report information and read or watch their stories.
- Understand the difference between news and advertising.
- Even if you are not included in the story, be patient and keep in touch with the writer.
- Understand that the media have a job to do. Help make their job easier by providing material in written form and give them what they ask for.
- Try to return calls or e-mails quickly. A late call back may result in losing your chance for a story.
- Designate a spokesperson in the clinic as a single point of contact for media.
- Contact only one person at the newspaper, radio, or television station to avoid duplication.
- Relate your story to the interests of your target audience and editorial needs of each outlet.

Optimized Press Releases

Once upon a time, press releases were called news releases and were used exclusively to announce milestones and newsworthy happenings. That tactic is so yesterday. In today's media-saturated climate, press releases are used for everything from new products, to clinic news, and to general information of no particular importance. Press releases have become a somewhat tired tool to drive readers to a website and social media channels.

From a media standpoint, press releases are one of the most overused web marketing tactics in the aesthetics industry. The Internet is flooded daily with a barrage of worthless press releases that are just not newsworthy. A common mistake is a failed attempt to craft a message around the interests of the reader rather than one's personal agenda. Does your audience really care about your clinic's new website? Are they truly interested in the fact that you have added a new machine/product/staff member? Probably not. They really only care about how your "news" will affect them. For example, does the new product solve a problem or answer an unmet need? Does it improve the user's quality of life? Is it better, faster, cheaper, easier, or improved over previous versions? If it does any of these things, lead with that angle instead of one that is more overtly self-serving.

Use the most important tidbit of information in the headline of the release and lead paragraph. Try to appeal to a specific target audience, and keep your key messages on point. Every paragraph and quote should support the key message you want to get across. It will help get your content in front of a larger audience and go live on other sites with hyperlinks in the content pointing back to the originating site.

Once you understand the keyword phrases that are both searched on and relevant, include them in the headline, subhead, and body of the release. Hyperlink the main keyword phrases you incorporate to a relevant page on your website. The link will be helpful for your search engine optimization (SEO) goals and will drive readers from the release to your website. Press releases can also incorporate images, video, and audio content to keep viewers engaged.

Although there are many free news release sites online, the best distribution services will ensure that your release reaches the most relevant channels for maximum results. These services also make it easy to tap into other tools and social media platforms. When drafted properly, press releases that are search engine optimization friendly can position your site to have higher search engine visibility.

Investing time and effort to optimize the content for your marketing materials is necessary to increase the number of readers who actually see your content and hopefully share it and bookmark it.

A press release posted to any social networking site can dramatically increase a news release's visibility. Users who click through news releases have an established interest in that subject area and are more likely to share the information with others. The collaborative nature of social media communities can amplify the reach and life of your releases.

HOW TO USE NEWS RELEASES

Spread the word about:

- New products, services
- Joint ventures, new partnerships
- Clinical research
- New divisions or subsidiaries
- Opinions on industry trends
- Survey results
- Events (open houses, speaking engagements)
- Personnel additions
- Volunteer work
- Milestones (years in business, awards)

New Rules for Releases

The purpose of a press release is to get your story in front of as many people as possible. Posting a release to a newswire service will distribute it to thousands of publications so it can get reposted by online outlets. They will also distribute releases directly to social media channels, especially Twitter, for broader reach. The more journalists who view your press release, the more pickup you may get. However, journalists literally get hundreds of press releases daily, so it is harder to stand out.

SEO-FRIENDLY PRESS RELEASE HEADLINES

- London Male Plastic Surgery Increases 50%
- Get Rid of Dimples and Cellulite without Cosmetic Surgery
- Women Opt for Natural Looking Breasts at Manchester Clinic
- New Mums Seek Non-Surgical Fat Melting for Post Baby Tummy
- Denver Plastic Surgeon Uses New Laser to Improve Burn Scars
- New Survey Shows More Women under 35 Consider Vein Treatments

Press releases are a lot less effective at generating media coverage today, especially in the era of social media. In fact, many will be deleted before they ever get read, particularly if the release was not targeted to the right media at the right time, or if it is poorly written. Before you send out a release, ask yourself if the information is remotely newsworthy. For example, consumer surveys, clinical study results, trend data, and case studies may be shared with media, and the media can actually use the information. Awards and milestones are fair game because they will elevate your clinic brand. Launching a new website or blog is definitely not of interest to the media, and these cheesy SEO tactics should be abandoned.

A compelling headline and well-crafted lead paragraph are the most critical things to get right. The opening paragraph should summarize your story succinctly to generate interest. Include a sharp subject line and visuals like photos and video clips so it will get noticed.

Digital Is the New Print

The pendulum has swung from print to online in terms of how people consume news, which has had a massive effect on the way media work. Journalists now use social media in their day-to-day hunt for great story ideas and expert sources.

More people get their news from digital sources and on their mobile devices. This represents a sea change in our consumption habits and explains why many magazines and newspapers have shut down their print editions. The majority of online outlets also have higher circulations than traditional print publications, so if you are keen to get "ink," do not only focus on print. Online placements will optimize your web presence and boost your search engine ranking. Print outlets have long lead times and cannot deliver the instant gratification consumers now demand. It can take months or even a year or more from the time you relay your message and connect with a journalist for the story to appear in print. Another plus is that online content lasts forever and is easy to recycle for social media.

A strong press release outlining why the topic is significant or interesting is key. The most effective releases tie into current news, announce a new treatment, or share a key industry development. Press releases and pitches can also attract the attention of bloggers who may have thousands of followers, which can catapult your clinic into the spotlight. You may also invite relevant local beauty influencers to trial some of the services you offer and spread the word through their own sphere of influence (see Chapter 8, section entitled "Influencer Marketing").

A journalist who covers a regular beat, such as health or beauty, will often be talking to the same people on a fairly regular basis. Actively participating in conversations on various platforms is the new normal way to forge relationships with sources that a journalist may not have otherwise come across. This especially helps when a journalist needs a source at the last minute. There will always be someone on Twitter or Facebook Messenger who will respond in record time to a query when a reporter is on deadline. Sources for stories almost always share the stories, and their audiences will often comment, which can lead to new story ideas.

To become a media darling, respecting deadlines is crucial. Writers are often on tight deadlines and will return to sources who respond in a timely manner and give them what they need. The preferred way editors want to reach sources are via e-mail, cell phone, text, or through their PR contact.

WENDYISM

Nothing is ever really off the record. You cannot retract something you said to the media and regretted later.

The media are not compelled to let you read the story before it goes to print. At best, you may have an opportunity to check your quotes. Few outlets have fact checkers or assistants anymore due to budget cuts. The sad truth is that most are operating on a skeleton crew, which is all the more reason to make their job easier if you want them to work with you.

Anything you say can show up in print, or be blogged about or tweeted, so never say anything that may not be in your best interest to share. Even if you state up front that your comments are "off the record," real reporters are not bound to abide by that request.

If you are serious about getting your name out there in the media, consider hiring a professional, beauty-savvy, connected publicist to guide you and help you stay out of trouble.

Patient Rewards Programs

Successful marketing strategies start and end with making patients a top priority. Patient acquisition adds growth opportunity, but the mainstay of your practice's longevity comes from loyal patients.

Reward patients for their referrals and loyalty by providing treatment vouchers, courtesy discounts, new product trials, sampling, and VIP status within your practice. Thank happy patients by showing them that you appreciate their business and referrals. They can become local brand ambassadors and spread the word about you.

Patients can be fickle as they are bombarded with a daily assault of deals for cheap laser hair removal and discounted filler injections. Rather than spending a fortune to constantly attract new patients, make taking special care of current patients a top priority. If a patient is satisfied with the experience in your clinic, he or she will return and hopefully refer friends. Acknowledging and rewarding patients who are loyal can go far to keep them.

Loyalty programs can be designed to offer perks ranging from access to appointment times, special pricing, invitations to private events, product samples, and introductory treatments. Consider implementing a VIP card with added benefits. For example, if you add a new laser, invite your VIP patients to come in for a complimentary trial. Offer an extra area of neurotoxin injection from time to time, or let them try a new skin care regime you are trialing for their feedback. These programs help patients become more consistent with their treatments. Make them feel special so they will stay with you.

Annual Marketing Plan

WENDYISM

Think of your marketing calendar as the bible you can refer to when any marketing decision needs to be made.

What is the difference between a "marketing strategy" and a "marketing plan?" Think of it this way— your marketing strategy should outline what your goals are, and your plan is all about how you are going to get there. Basically, you cannot have one without the other. It is not the same as your marketing calendar; rather it is an integral part of it.

A detailed, well-structured 12-month marketing calendar will serve as the road map to marketing prowess—that is, if you stick to it. Start by breaking down the year by quarters, then by months, and then by weeks. Address all of the main marketing activities that will take place during each period, and as many of the smaller projects as possible. Spell out general marketing programs first, and then add more detail by itemizing individual promotions or events when the information has been finalized. The more specific your marketing calendar is, the better it will work. Set up reminders for all deadlines for insertion orders, art requirements, e-blasts to be sent, and so on, to stay on top of every activity.

For example, you may be bringing in a new piece of capital equipment, which could be your focus for the quarter. You can next decide how to promote it on a month-by-month basis. The first month may include an introduction to your VIP patients with a private reception where they are encouraged to bring a friend, and an e-blast to announce that you have something new to offer. For month two, you may run an ad campaign in your local newspaper's website. For the third month, you can promote the new treatment with a geo-targeted Facebook and Instagram ad campaign.

Whereas a strategic marketing plan integrates long-term planning (3–5 years) and short-term implementation, a marketing calendar is a short-term plan that itemizes the immediate day-to-day implementation of individual tactics. At a more tactical level, an annual marketing calendar should dovetail with your long-term strategic marketing plan to ensure that every action is geared toward achieving your strategic goals. The best time to address your marketing calendar is toward the end of the year to start fresh at the beginning of a new year. Plan to reflect on what worked and what did not, and what you want to do differently next year. For best results, make it a team effort and get the whole clinic involved in the process.

5 REASONS WHY YOU NEED A MARKETING CALENDAR

1. To stay organized

An annual marketing calendar organizes the tactics to help you launch marketing programs, campaigns, and initiatives throughout the year in a way that forces you to stay on track. It will assist you in figuring out what you need to do and when to do it for maximum impact. Ideally, if you follow the marketing calendar you created (optimally to start January 1 for the year), you can capitalize on every opportunity to market your practice without any lapses. Your planning, budgeting, staffing, and consultants will be handled. Within your calendar, you may also delegate a separate, detailed daily social media calendar for blogs and all content for your practice social channels that coordinates with the main marketing calendar.

2. To stay on track

A marketing calendar crystallizes your focus and allows you to analyze the investment and value of your marketing tactics to help build consistency into your planning. You can avoid that feeling of panic that sets in when the phone stops ringing or patient visits slow down. The time to jump-start your marketing tactics is not when business is slow. By fleshing out a calendar, you can plan well in advance for the slower months.

Aesthetic medicine is not always cyclical; however, certain months are naturally busier than others. For example, the fourth quarter is prime time for procedures and noninvasive treatments due to the holidays, family gatherings, and special events. January is a notoriously quiet month. Summer can be slow, but August can be active if your practice attracts specific segments of customers, such as students, teachers, and therapists who may have time off at the end of summer. In some markets, the winter or summer season is when the population swells from the arrival of visitors and tourists. When drafting a marketing calendar, keep in mind what your best months are and when your practice is at risk of slowing down. Take into account all the factors that could affect your business.

3. To enable clear decision making

Having determined the critical success factors that affect your clinic, and deciding on the resources you have to deal with them, you are in a better position to make smarter marketing decisions. Are your services meeting your customers' needs, or should you add new treatments? Is your pricing strategy right for the market? Do you need extra staff or should you outsource marketing or social media services? Do you need PR or a bigger budget for SEO? The questions that arise will be easier to navigate in the context of a marketing calendar with clear timing, planning, and budget. It will also help defer reactive decisions by providing the framework to make sound choices. You will know what is set up for the next months and weeks, and are less likely to make decisions on the fly in response to market developments or external pressures from vendors.

4. To manage your budget

Create a marketing budget to make it easy to see at a glance which events and strategies were productive and on target, and delivered the best ROI. This will aid you in planning for future periods. Each year you should revisit your marketing calendar template and revise it accordingly. Your next marketing calendar should reflect changes and additions based on the previous year. For example, if your monthly Facebook advertising budget delivered positive results, you may want to increase that budget going forward. But if you ran an ad series in a local magazine that did not generate enough patients to pay for itself, you can redirect that budget to something else.

5. Because shift happens

Think of your marketing calendar as a working document; plan to make changes and additions along the way. New issues may arise at any time that may call for a deviation in strategy. A regular review will reveal what you have followed and completed, results that were tracked, and any holes. How frequently you revisit your calendar will depend on the nature of your practice and the extent to which the factors affecting it change. For example, a new treatment that gains U.S. Food and Drug Administration clearance that you want to offer in your clinic may necessitate a change in strategy. You may decide to take budget from one quarter and move it up or push it to the next month.

MONTHLY MARKETING CALENDAR TEMPLATE

Month

	Activity	Date Scheduled	Team Member	Materials Needed	Due Dates	Vendor(s)	Cost	Results	Next Steps
Week 1									
Week 2									
Week 3									
Week 4									

WHAT GOES INTO A MARKETING CALENDAR

- Major holidays and seasonal events
- Local/regional events (health fairs, charity benefits, parades, garden shows, etc.)
- National events (sports, news stories, celebrities, etc.)
- Award shows (Emmys, Oscars, BAFTAs, etc.)
- Disease-specific dates (skin cancer, breast cancer, etc.)
- Social media events (Throwback Thursday, Fitness Friday, Sunday Funday)
- Speaking engagements
- "Hallmark holidays" (National Lipstick Day, etc.)

To find out any dates that may be relevant for your clinic, visit daysoftheyear.com

3

Clinic Website—The Marketing Mothership

The aim of marketing is to know and understand the customer so well the product or service fits him and sells itself.

Peter Drucker

WENDYISM

Your clinic website is your marketing mothership.

In today's digital world, having a dedicated website for your practice is a critical component of giving patients instant access to information about your practice, special expertise, and the products and services you offer.

An informative and interactive website with the right updated content will strongly position your practice as being committed to delivering the highest level of patient care and education. Patients today go online more than ever to research and gather knowledge about health and well-being. By having a website that can be easily found on search engines, with relevant, consumer-friendly content, you can stand out against your competitors and consistently attract new patients.

Basic search engine optimization strategies go a long way toward increasing the visibility of your site. By customizing your site with the specific products and treatments you offer, coupled with compelling before and after images, patients will be able to find what they are looking for in a few clicks, and make informed decisions regarding their own treatment.

Strive to design or update your site with fresh content on a regular basis—monthly for some categories and weekly or biweekly for special offers, blog posts, events, and so on. Create an inviting, aesthetically pleasing site that uses proven strategies people are seeking, such as a photo gallery, blog entries, special promotions, and downloadable educational brochures about your clinic and procedures, as well as pre- and postprocedural instructions.

Web marketing (now called digital marketing) is the most highly effective, efficient, and affordable means of driving patients to your practice. When done well and consistently, it provides the best return on investment (ROI), bar none.

Staying on Brand

Having an updated and optimized website today is a mandatory initiative for all successful aesthetic clinics, and your website should be created to reflect the personality and positioning of your clinic. Patients are searching for local businesses online, so your site must be optimized for search engine pickup. If it isn't, only people searching for you by name will find your clinic online.

Promoting your clinic is no longer only about having a pretty brochure or an adequate website. You also need to be present in all the other places where your patients go, live, read, and play. Marketing your clinic now is about creating multiple touch points to connect with your target audience in meaningful ways.

Think Mobile Friendly

With the advent of advanced mobile devices becoming a fact of life across all demographics, mobile marketing has taken center stage. If your website is not searchable on mobile platforms, you are unwittingly turning visitors away. It is important to be readable on thumb-friendly mobile platforms because the majority of your website's traffic will come from phones and other mobile devices. So, if your website is not easy to navigate, clickable or legible on a tiny screen, you are missing out on capturing the attention of most of your prospective patients.

Since the screen size of a mobile phone or tablet is small, the scope of content that can be displayed is limited. The best content for mobile devices, whether it is text, images, or video, needs to be a lot simpler than for desktops or laptops. At a minimum, your website should have the capability of being viewed on a small screen at least the size of an iPad mini and preferably an iPhone or Android phones. Reaching out to patients on the technology they use offers many unique benefits, including lower costs, improved customization, easier tracking, and reduced staff time.

Creating a mobile version of your practice website is a worthwhile investment. It does not have to cost a fortune to convert your existing website to a mobile-friendly version. If you are designing a new website, use "responsive design" to make it look good on all screens from the get go.

Above the Fold

> **Remember when being "social" meant going to someone's home? Now it is more like going to someone's home page.**

The top of the landing page of any website contains the most valuable real estate.

You have only three seconds to convince visitors that your site is worth any more of their time. Therefore, the look and feel of your site should create the desired effect.

The landing page should contain the words or pictures that are already on the minds of your target audience, and it should deliver on any promise your external marketing program makes for consistency. The top of the landing page—above the fold—should contain the most important details. Tell visitors who you are, what you do, where you are located, and how to reach you by including a phone number, e-mail link, and/or scheduling form.

ESSENTIAL ELEMENTS OF A GREAT LANDING PAGE

- Clinic credentials—Certification, specialty
- Location—Neighborhood, city, state or province
- Call to action—Scheduling form, e-mail contact, phone
- Testimonials—From patients, media
- Reviews/links
- Trust symbols—Organizations, brands, affiliations, awards
- Photo(s)—Doctor, staff, facility
- Map/navigation—How to find you
- Key services—What do you offer?
- Photo gallery—Section most visited by consumers
- All social buttons

Every landing page needs a clear call to action (CTA)—a message that tells visitors what to do next. For example, having a "Contact Us" form for patients to fill out and submit for more information will help you capture inbound patient information for future follow-up and to add to your database. Another example is a readily displayed phone number to schedule an appointment. These should be prominently placed so visitors don't have to scroll to find them. Place a "Contact Us" link near the top of every page throughout the site. Another example of a creative CTA would be a call-out on the landing page a complimentary consultation for a new service.

Components of a Killer Website

Web content is one thing clinic managers have control over, so do not overload your site with excessive nonessential or irrelevant text. The motivation is understandable—your website is the hub of your online marketing presence; you want to share everything you can about your clinic and make sure your keywords are included in your text. This strategy can be a detriment to functionality as users can get lost in pages of text, or may be turned off by too many clicks to get to what they want to read. Since the attention span of users is so short, text should be short and to the point.

Your site should have two primary goals: to provide brand awareness and to generate new customers. Keeping your content short and to the point will inspire customers to contact you. Landing page content should be easy to read and understand and tell the story that is on your visitors' minds. Show how your products and services help a potential patient. Use words and phrases they would use to describe the problems they want to solve.

Keeping text brief on the landing page makes it clear and uncluttered and helps people understand what you are saying quickly. It also downloads and performs faster, giving users a better experience so they will stay on the site longer and convert to customers more often. Do not be afraid of some white space.

Showcase Your Skills

A curriculum vitae (CV) is much more than a résumé for physicians. It serves as a record of a lifelong accumulation of milestones, training, degrees, and accomplishments and follows your career from your undergraduate experience through to retirement. Therefore, do not expect anyone to take the time to read through every research project you did in medical school or conference attended. In many cases, these additional facts will just dilute the most important highlights you want to convey.

Aesthetic physicians should maintain a consumer-friendly bio that includes the accolades they are programmed to look for in priority order (i.e., most important first). It may be useful to have several versions at the ready for different purposes; a one-paragraph biographical description of under 250 words, as well as a brief bio of your expertise.

ELEMENTS OF A CONSUMER-FRIENDLY BIO

- Name and degree
- Board certification or other qualifications
- Areas of specialization
- Media recognition
- Honors and awards
- Current hospital appointments
- Academic positions or professional titles
- Relevant professional memberships
- Education (graduate, fellowships, training)

Include a brief narrative followed by bullets of key details. A full CV can be added as a link to a separate page or downloadable PDF. Focus on major professional accomplishments, education, and training. It should be concise and deliver the message that you are qualified and have the requisite expertise to leave the visitor wanting to know more about you. To personalize it, add a quote in the first person that expresses your philosophy about aesthetics, medicine, or patient-centric care.

Your photo should be current, taken in the last 3 years at maximum. If you had a full head of dark hair once, and have a sparse head of gray hair now, you will look very different to patients when they first meet you, which can be misleading. A personal video introduction on the landing page is a welcome addition to make patients feel comfortable with you before they come to the clinic.

Site Navigation

Navigation is how visitors go from page to page or section to section of the site and how they find what they are looking for. There are three basic ways to navigate a website. It is recommended to implement all three navigation types throughout your site for a consistent user experience:

1. Horizontal navigation (across the top)
2. Vertical navigation (usually on the left side)
3. Footer (at the bottom of each page)

Web surfers have short attention spans, and they will not spend extra time on a site if they cannot find their way around easily. Place the navigation where users expect to find it—either across the top horizontally or on the left as a vertical sidebar—and place the navigation menus in the same location on every page for consistency. Maintain the same style, fonts, and colors throughout the site, and do not go too crazy. By following these simple design principles, users will get used to the style of the site and the look and feel of your brand. As they get comfortable, they will (hopefully) spend more time browsing, which is the ultimate goal.

Use phrases in your navigation that are specific. Avoid vague terms like "News" or "Resources." These can be left open to interpretation. Choose terms that are clear and three words or less, such as "Patient Gallery," "About Our Clinic," and "Meet Our Doctors." Make it easy for users to find what they are looking for in under three clicks. If it takes more than that, they may give up and leave the site in frustration.

Think about what you like and do not like about the sites you visit. Does the page load quickly? Is it easy to get where you want to go? Are there any "Page Not Found" notifications popping up?

Less Is More

Site navigation and organization are key components of effective search engine optimization, so if you want to be found by Google, be specific. A good number of links to consider for your menus is six or eight items maximum. Do not overwhelm users with too many choices that can cause confusion. Drop-down menus can be used for more specific terms, but these may not get picked up by search engines.

Make sure you have a visible link on each page so the reader can get back to a previous page or the home page quickly to keep it user friendly.

The footer is the series of links that appear at the very bottom of the site's landing page. This area contains technical information, including copyright and date, name of the site's owner, business name and address, links to key pages within the website, and an e-mail link.

Photo Gallery

One picture is worth a thousand words.

Fred R. Barnard

We live in a very visual age where pictures draw more attention than words.

A robust photo gallery of actual patients to showcase your results is usually the section that consumers go to first. If you do not have good photographs to post, your site will be at a supreme disadvantage. It is important to avoid blacked-out eyes, pictures of facial regions instead of the entire face, and blurry photos with bad lighting or inconsistent angles, or makeup, too much hair on the face, and jewelry. Consumers are very wise to the tricks of photo enhancing, so if your photos do not ring true, they may be suspicious. Descriptors let visitors know exactly what treatment was performed and the interval between the before and after photos. Wherever possible, select photos that match the target audience to which you are marketing. For example, if you are targeting men, a page of photos of women is not relevant to that audience.

I strongly recommend watermarking all patient photos you post online so they are less likely to be lifted and end up on Facebook or RealSelf or another clinic's website. Remember that patient photos require written consent from the patient that should be kept on file in their chart, and this consent can be rescinded at any time.

Microsite Marketing

A microsite allows you focus on a specific purpose, such as promoting a treatment or category of treatments such as "body contouring," or featuring your special expertise in a specific area, such as "vaginal rejuvenation" or treating a unique group of patients, such as men. The design and navigation of a microsite may differ from your main site, but it does not have to. Ideally it should compliment rather than just duplicate your main site to set your microsite apart. Microsite marketing can be an effective technique to drive additional visitors to your site. The concept of developing microsites specifically targeted to new segments of potential clients allows your practice to establish a broader presence online among niche markets.

But there are pros and cons to this strategy, as Google's search algorithm tends to reward trusted, well-established domains and unique content. A microsite may risk diluting your brand and hurting your search results in some cases. However, the benefits may outweigh the risks if you want to create a targeted, strategic marketing campaign.

A microsite is basically an edited selection of web pages that are differentiated from a parent or main website through unique design and layout, limited navigation options, and a unique domain name or URL. These can also be used to promote specialized, short-term offers or new product launches, but the main advantage is to attract new segments of patients and customers. A microsite focuses on a specific area, such as promoting your services for a particular procedure like breast enhancement, or on a specific group of consumers, like those seeking mommy makeovers. They are intended to target only one area of your practice, usually a procedure in which you specialize, or a specific geographic location, or a patient group from which you would like to attract more clients.

Microsites may be used to focus on in-depth information about a narrower area of specialization with a unique visitor experience. The microsites will be linked to your main site, so they can create better traffic from all the online sources to your main website. Because a microsite is often designed to target one primary search term, it can move quickly up the search engine rank for the primary term you select. Typically, a microsite will mirror similar branding, imagery, and design of the main site. In some cases, the design and navigation may need to differ slightly from your main site to attract a different audience entirely.

One commonly used example is to market to a specific ethnic group of potential patients, such as Spanish-speaking patients or patients from the Middle East. In this case, it may be wise to develop a microsite that is linked to the landing page of your main site, as well as build a unique URL for that page (e.g., xyzclinic.com and xyzclinicenespanol.com).

12 POPULAR MICROSITE THEMES

- Skin of color
- Breast enhancement
- Body contouring
- International patients
- Spanish-speaking patients or any other language
- Cosmetic procedures for men
- Acne treatments
- Hair restoration
- Millennials
- Vaginal rejuvenation
- Mommy makeover
- Skincare/spa treatments

A microsite strategy can be effectively combined with your search campaigns so that as your microsite gains rankings in search engines, it begins to take on organic links and establish a greater presence for your clinic. Along with the added value of your microsite, your main site gains additional value in the form of referral traffic and optimized links. Instead of depending on one complex megasite to feature content about everything you offer, the option of increasing your footprint on search engines offers another way to attract more clients.

Microsites can be just a few pages, so they are affordable compared to an overhaul of your main website and can be created in less time. Microsite marketing can be a rewarding strategy to add and a worthwhile investment when designed with your specific goals and endgame in mind.

A microsite enables you to position yourself as an expert in a specific procedure category. Visitors will most likely find your microsite while looking for a specific procedure in your geographic location, they are considered highly qualified. By providing valuable procedure-specific information, a related photo gallery, and unique videos and content, visitors will identify your practice as a leader in the field.

Another option is to have a few larger sites for specialized areas that contain a steady supply of updated content. For example, you may want to identify two or three key areas of your practice that are worth investing in to grow. These might include categories where there is less competition in your market to allow for a higher return.

Look for domain names that have popular search phrases used by potential customers. Consider how consumers will use the web to search for the procedure you are marketing (e.g., HairrestorationUK.com or BreastliftsMiami.com). Domain names can be chosen based on keyword research to determine which would yield the best traffic from the major search engines. Another commonly used strategy is to create a microsite for nonsurgical or skincare and spa services that is linked to your main site, which may focus on more invasive procedures. Many practitioners also maintain a microsite that contains a shopping cart for their own branded skincare or cosmetic line.

Whatever you decide, make sure the strategy has been well researched for validation, and that it will not dilute your marketing budget by stealing valuable traffic from your main bread-and-butter site.

4

Web Marketing from Soup to Nuts

There are no secrets to success. It is the result of preparation, hard work, and learning from failure.

Colin Powell

As soon as you think you are up to date on the latest Google algorithm or Facebook conspiracy, something unexpected will always come around the corner to throw you off your game. Google changes its search algorithm over 500 times every year. While most of these changes are minor, every few months they roll out a major algorithmic update that affects search results in significant ways.

If you are not paying attention to these updates, it is easy to get confused and frustrated. As search engines update and change their algorithms, some tactics you may have adopted a few years or even months ago may no longer be relevant today and can potentially be hurting you. You need to enlist the services of a credible web marketing team you can trust to stay on top of it all.

The primary goal of Google and other leading search engines is to provide the best possible answers to the queries of the searchers. Therefore, the search engine would ideally rank a website that provides the best information for a reader's query on top of the search results. Search engine spiders are not looking for websites with the best search engine optimization (SEO) techniques, but those websites with the best and most relevant content that addresses a searcher's query.

Google's methods are aimed at weeding out sites that operate just to outsmart search engine spiders, rather than focusing on providing good and original content. Google has made its search algorithm more comprehensive by adding more weight to social media activity and what they consider to be high-quality back links. This helps to identify the best sites to give them top search engine ranking so they appear first.

If You Build It…

> **WENDYISM**
>
> *When it comes to websites, the adage, "If you build it, they will come" does not apply.*

In today's competitive environment, a website is the lifeline to your practice, much like the phone system used to be. It has become a virtual necessity for all physicians offering elective services. Think of your website as an electronic brochure. Unlike expensive glossy brochures, there is a greater opportunity for potential patients to view your website and react to the information.

Just having a site is only one part of the equation. Beyond the basics of SEO and PPC (Pay-Per-Click) or paid ads, your digital strategy may include participating in online forums, asking patients to post reviews, engaging in social media, e-mail marketing, building links, and much more. Web-based marketing is the single, most cost-effective way for practitioners to increase their presence and credibility online and to get their message across to attract new patients.

Search Engine Optimization Best Practices

Do not try this at home. SEO is a complex process that changes often. Therefore, it is vital to consult with a professional web developer or agency to help you optimize your site. This is not something you want to just experiment with, because chances are you will get it wrong and will have to start all over again.

SEO is an ongoing process of improving your website and earning links from other relevant sites. The overriding goal of SEO is to get your site ranked in the top positions of organic search results for the keywords relevant to your product, brand, or services.

You can be visible on search engines in two ways: PPC and SEO. The benefits of SEO are different than those of paid search. In essence, paid search results are bought, and organic search results are earned. In some ways, it is like the difference between editorial and advertising. Editorial coverage is earned (meaning you are not paying the publication to write about you), whereas advertising is strictly pay for play.

To understand SEO, the goal is to get your site ranked in the top positions of organic search results for the keywords relevant to your clinic. To determine the right keywords, you need to put yourself in the minds of your potential customers. What are they searching for so you can lead them to your site? Keyword selection has a lot to do with understanding who your target customer is.

Unlike paid search where you can add multiple keywords and let the marketplace determine which ones drive the most traffic to your site, SEO requires a lot of effort to rank for each keyword you choose, so you need to choose those keywords with great care.

Search engines use automated spiders (or bots) to crawl and index the web. This is how they know that sites exist and what content they contain. So, if your site is not set up properly to allow these spiders to crawl through your content, the content will not get found or have a chance of being ranked.

Think the Way Consumers Think

Well-optimized content has to be of good quality so that people want to read it. Focus on your target audience, and address the questions, concerns, and needs they may have about your products and services. Provide your content in a visually pleasing manner, using images, headings, and subheadings, to make it simple to read. You need to have enough content to include all of the keywords that you have selected to rank. You can target multiple related keywords (up to five is a good range) on a page, and a page for each major keyword you want to target. Those pages should also follow certain best practices, such as including the keyword in the title tag, once in a header tag, and then two to three times in the page content.

Research keywords and back your choices with data about search volume related to those keywords, and you should end up with a keyword portfolio that will drive traffic to your site as if it were ranked in the top three for all of your terms. Google AdWords Keyword Planner is a helpful free tool. Make sure your site is search-engine friendly, so that the spiders can crawl and index it, and develop unique content around the keywords you need. If you dedicate enough effort and budget to build the right links to your site from the right places, you can eventually rank at the top of the search engines.

Organic Searches

Organic search results are not paid for. These are the listings that come up first when specific keywords are entered by the user. If your listing does not pop up on the first page for the keywords that really count for your clinic, the most valuable consumers may not be able to find you unless they are searching for you by name. Like paid search, a viable SEO strategy is a critical tool for driving new patients to your site.

Organic search listings are considered to be unbiased endorsements of the ranked sites. Searchers view organic search results as the best option according to the all-knowing search engines. This drives trust for your brand that can go a long way toward winning customers.

The traffic you get from organic search results is free, because you do not pay for each click on your listing as you do with PPC. However, a lot of time, money, and effort can go into getting your site to rank well in organic search. Organic search can account for a substantial amount of traffic over that of paid search.

Content Is King

WENDYISM

Don't take the lazy doctor's way out. Create original meaningful content that speaks to your target audience and elevates your brand.

The focus of search engines on the actual content on a page makes the job of the person entrusted with creating the content even more important. Arguably, the content plays the most significant role in generating good results. As Google states, "Make pages primarily for users, not for search engines."

The most popular content that gets to the top of the search engine results page has several qualities worth noting. Generally, it has been deemed to be more useful and interesting than other content. Another Google proviso is to ask yourself, "Does this help my users?" and "Would I do this if search engines did not exist?" Perhaps if we all followed this mantra, there would be a lot less white noise out there to plow through on a daily basis.

Optimizing content now is harder than before. It requires you to consider what your target audience is interested in knowing more about. It is not just about throwing in a string of keywords into your copy and posting it. SEO tactics focus less on technical aspects and instead are focused on user experience. The best kind of content earns credibility when real people actually read, use, and share it throughout their own social networks. Search engines really like content that gets talked about, commented on, and liked, and tend to reward the original poster accordingly.

The most effective sites contain 100% unique content, which is what draws visitors. If the information is readily available everywhere else on the web, visitors have no reason to come to your site and stay. Even if your web marketing drives traffic to the site, the lack of original content of interest to the visitor may cause visitors to log out in a few seconds and move on to another site. Therefore, the more distinctive and original content, in your own voice, that appears on your websites and blog, the better results you can achieve.

Lifting content from the sites of professional organizations and vendors whose equipment or products you offer is risky business. Similarly, adopting content you find online from random informational sites, Wikipedia, About.com, and others, should be discouraged. If search engines find the same text on your blog, press releases, or website that appears everywhere else, it will most likely be ignored. But if your content is unique, interesting, and of high quality, you have a better chance of ranking higher among leading search engines. In addition, better content attracts more traffic and incoming links, which in turn, also help your ranking with the search engines.

The more generic and uninspired your content is, the less readable it will be to visitors; therefore, it is less likely to be seen by the audiences you are targeting—search engines as well as patients. Duplicate content generally refers to blocks of content that are either identical or extremely similar. Maintaining a good balance of unique with duplicate content will allow you to stay under the radar of the almighty Google and other search engines.

As some of us know firsthand, the wrath of Google is not fun. If Google determines that you are deliberately plugging in duplicated content to manipulate search engine rankings or gain more traffic, it may be considered deceptive and therefore a violation. Google's mission is to index and show pages with distinct information to offer users a rich experience. Therefore, if you have low-quality, generic content, you are at risk. Defying Google leaves you vulnerable to penalties, which can manifest in many ways. It is possible to have your site's organic rankings significantly decline or in extreme cases the site will be taken down for days, weeks, or even longer, which, in effect, can strangle your business especially if you rely heavily on your web presence to attract new patients.

Each page of your site should be unique, even if it is similar to the theme of another page. Avoid lifting content directly from other sites, such as procedural descriptions from professional organizations or information from vendors' sites whose products you use. This is the lazy doctor's way to create a website. Everything you add to your site should be customized and reflect the personal style or voice of the physician and the practice. Each page of your site has value; you do not want to populate your pages with content that may undermine your overall mission of driving more traffic. Your site should be uniquely yours, and not just a duplication of every other cosmetic surgeon's site.

Search engines attempt to filter their search results by removing any results that duplicate the content of other search. To avoid using duplicate content, make sure that your content is written exclusively for your use and that you own the copyright. Include a copyright notice in the footer, for example, ©*2018 John Smith, MD, PC.*

Even if pages on your site look very different in terms of colors, order of words, layout, design, or graphics, search engines will only detect differences if the content is dramatically different. If there is an instance where you need to use duplicate content, such as referencing a news item or sharing a blog post, also add unique content. If there is more unique content than duplicate content, the risk of having the page flagged by search engines is reduced.

DUPLICATE CONTENT FIX

If you have concerns that you may have duplicate content, perform a site check on www.copyscape. com. Enter the URL of the page, and it will return a list of pages Google has indexed that contain text that is duplicated on your site. Rewrite any duplicate copy so that search engines can reindex the page with new, original content.

Working with a web marketing agency that does not have strong copywriting skills or direct knowledge of the field of aesthetic medicine is risky and can work to your disadvantage.

Choosing Keywords

Keyword research is at the core of SEO. To improve your search visibility, you must identify the phrases that are used most often and incorporate phrases that users are searching for regularly. For example, using descriptive words along with your clinic name will create your identity online and allow visitors to find you based on their interests. Look at phrases or variations that Google lists as additional options. Find out which are the most commonly used terms for the energy-based devices or dermal fillers you offer. Expand your list further by including brand and product names, and your geographical area. Using an edited list of keywords, work closely with a web designer on page headlines, subheadlines, and opening paragraphs for each page that include these words and phrases.

Set a reasonable budget for what you want to achieve in terms of site visitors, new patients, and increased revenue, and for engaging a firm that has good references and wide experience working in the medical space. Think of search terms consumers will use to find the treatments you want to promote. Focus on the most profitable treatments first, rather than trying to be everywhere. For example, if someone is looking for a specific topic, such as "cellulite reduction," you want your site to be as high up on search engines as you can afford so patients can land there. Pay-Per-Click (PPC) Adverts are an integral part of a web marketing program. These are the ads you see on the top area of Google's results pages and at the bottom, below organic placements.

Search engines such as Google, Yahoo!, and Bing have programs in place that search for the most relevant content for any given keyword. Therefore, it is important to ensure that the main keywords you selected are used often in the content and are also tagged on the page name. Best recommendations include targeting three to five main keywords or phrases on each page, and ensuring that each of your keywords is repeated at least two or three times in your page copy.

**EXAMPLES OF KEYWORDS SEARCHED BY CONSUMERS
SEEKING AESTHETIC TREATMENTS**

- Skin rejuvenation
- Laser skin resurfacing
- Wrinkle reducing treatments
- Nonsurgical facelift
- Skin tightening laser
- Acne treatments for teens
- Breast enhancement surgery
- Facial fillers before and after
- Best skin lightening treatment
- Nonsurgical bodyshaping
- Fat reduction laser
- Facial fillers

For tips on how to build the best keyword list, see google.com/adwords/.

Link Building

Buliding backlinks is a vital component of a digital marketing strategy. By definition, a backlink is an incoming hyperlink from one website to another.

Anytime a website mentions your name, brand, or company name with a link to your site, that is called a "backlink" and these are worth their weight in gold. Getting mentioned and linked to from other sites will increase traffic to your page to get your content and site in front or more eyes.

To increase your site's search engine results, increase the number of other sites that you link to or connect to from your website, for example, tags or icon links directly to your Facebook business page, Twitter account, and YouTube channel, and also including your URL (website address) when sending out any digital campaigns such as e-blasts, e-books, and so on.

Links (inbound links, back links, or external links) are an important factor that influences a site's search engine rankings. The spiders that crawl the web will never even find your site if there are no links pointing to it. Another valid reason to have inbound links is that they help to show search engines how popular your site is, and each link increases your popularity. The more links your site has compared to your competition, the higher its chance is to rank well.

Link building is a difficult and time-consuming SEO function, and all links are not created equal. Everything from the page and site from which you get your link, down to the text that is used in that link, provides different levels of value to your site. It is more than just a simple numbers game when it comes to links because of all of these nuances. Typically, the higher-quality links are the most difficult to obtain. The higher the quality of content you have, the easier your link-building task will be. In addition, other site owners are more likely to provide a link to your site if it provides quality content in a well-designed manner.

BACKLINK 5-POINT ACTION PLAN

1. Fix broken links that can harm your site's ranking.
2. Write guest posts on other sites to get a backlink to your own site.
3. Check out what your competitors are doing via https://monitorbacklinks.com/.
4. Be active about promoting your content by sharing blog posts, and via social media.
5. Comment on relevant articles, blogs, industry, and consumer sites to get noticed.

Local Searches

Consumers are turning to their mobile devices to find nearby businesses. To make sure your clinic can be found, include the street address, zip code, phone number, and other towns or cities you attract patients from on every page of your site. Create a free listing for your clinic on Google, Yahoo!, and Bing so that it shows up on a map when potential patients do a local search.

Local searchers are most often looking for products and services that they need relatively quickly compared to other searchers. For example, a consumer might see an ad for CoolSculpting on televsion or read a company advert in a magazine for a new filler, and instantly want to find out who is offering in their area. For potential patients to know that you are in their area, they first have to see your information in their search results. This is where SEO comes in to alert consumers that your local business offers services that matter to them. Online local searching can play a big role in driving consumers to buy products and choose one clinic over another.

Google Ads

Google and Bing PPC ads are among the most effective ways of driving to your site, specifically when people are searching for the products or services your clinic features. These ads appear in search results alongside non-paid (organic) results. Display Ads, mostly banners which appear on the Google Display Network, appear on millions of sites that have partnered with Google to sell ad space on their behalf. Google ads on the Display Network can be in the form of text, image, animation, or video.

In essence, the Google AdWords auction allows you to select a list of keywords to target that are relevant to your business. These are the words that people are most likely to use when searching for what you offer. Bid on these keywords by setting a fee for what you are willing to spend for each Google user to click on your ad. The cost varies based on many factors, including how competitive your keywords are, industry, location, and the quality of your ad campaign. For example, to buy a very common keyword in a major market where the competition is high, such as "Non-Surgical Body Shaping NYC," you have to be prepared to spend a lot more than the same keyword for less-crowded markets, like "Non-Surgical Body Shaping Nova Scotia."

Remarketing Program

Without remarketing, prospective patients may visit your site once and never come back. Remarketing strategically markets and targets visitors to your practice website with advertisements as they browse other popular websites. This strategy keeps your clinic in front of potentially viable patients and it can be highly effective. Remarketing can be a very useful strategy to get your clinic in front of more targeted eyes. This refers to techniques used by digital marketers to follow up with website visitors who do not conclude an action on the site such as to make a purchase, book an appointment, or fill out a contact form. Think about the last time you left something in your shopping cart without checking out. Did you all of a sudden feel like that brand was stalking you all over the web because a banner ad kept popping up? This strategy aims to bring visitors back to the site to convert them to making a purchase or signing up for a newsletter or whatever call to action (CTA) you feature. A remarketing campaign can be a useful source of new leads for your clinic. This is how remarketing works and it can be better than other digital ads, in terms of Cost Per Lead (CPL).

Your brand will be consistently promoted to consumers which can lead to a high conversion rate. As visitors continuously see your brand's key messages as they surf online, the more they become aware of your brand. Recognition equals trust, which equals higher conversion.

Google+: The Forgotten Platform

Google+ is primarily good for SEO and content sharing; after all, it is owned by Google. Sharing to Google+ can be tedious, and users never seemed to be very passionate about this platform. You do not hear or read much about it anymore, although it is still powerful.

If you are on the fence about whether Google+ is worth your time and what its true value is, consider these thoughts on why it is still relevant. Because Google basically ranks their own social network higher, your content on Google+ is more likely to show up in search results than other content because the decks are clearly stacked in their favor.

To participate in Google+, you need to build a network of Google+ circles. The more people you add to circles and the more people who add you to their circles, the more likely you are to show up high in search results. To take advantage of this strategy, make sure that your Google+ profile and page are complete so that Google can index them. Do not give up on Google+ just yet—it still has value for your clinic's digital footprint.

TIPS FOR USING GOOGLE+

- Go to your Google+ personal profile, and hit "Edit Profile."
- Click the "I" icon to go to the About Me page.
- Add your Introduction using words that relate to your brand in your tagline and About section.
- Make sure your Introduction is set to Public.
- Click on the + at the bottom of the page to include links to your sites and blog.
- Own your custom URL with your full clinic name.
- Share content including blog posts actively to get ranked.
- Keep building your Google+ circles.

5

Your Online Reputation

A passionate belief in your business and personal objectives can make all the difference between success and failure. If you aren't proud of what you're doing, why should anybody else be?

Richard Branson

Consumers can rate almost everything online today: books, salons, florists, hotels, restaurants—and even doctors. Whereas reviews for hotels tend to focus on location, amenities, comfort, and price, doctor ratings often focus on a long list of issues that are more subjective. These may include waiting times, scheduling snafus, décor, fees, and bedside manner, often more than the results and outcomes of treatments and services.

The landscape of aesthetic medicine has changed radically. Patients are more plugged in and command a high level of electronic connectivity from their healthcare providers. Aesthetic patients are also more demanding, have high expectations, and all too frequently change their doctors and go clinic shopping, for many reasons, including better service, lower costs, location, likeability, long wait times, billing errors, and staff changes.

Without a doubt, the decks are stacked against practitioners because they are greatly limited in how they can respond to public posts. Online interactions with patients about their medical treatment and care in your clinic, such as e-mail exchanges, are widely accepted. However, these conversations should never occur on a social networking platform or open forum.

The idea of online reputation and reviews is relatively new to medicine, but it is rapidly taking on increasing importance. Social media and online reviews are now considered critical success factors for aesthetic practitioners as well as all medical practices in light of the new consumer behavior and the value reviews have taken on. They are crucial tools for keeping your practice on the cutting edge.

Monitoring Your Brand Online

Relying solely on word-of-mouth marketing just will not cut it anymore. You need to reach new patients where they are. Review and rating sites rely on public information to populate their profiles, and your profile will exist whether you initiate it or not. In fact, you need to be vigilant because in many cases, public information is wrong or outdated, and the range of possible errors is vast. Your clinic may be mislabeled or categorized incorrectly, the name may be spelled wrong, qualifications may be incorrect, and even the location may be wrong. All of these errors can result in lost patients and a slump in revenue through no fault of your own.

7 ESSENTIAL STEPS TO CHECK YOUR ONLINE REPUTATION

1. Find and own your online listings on all relevant top rating and review sites within and outside of your market.
2. Update and complete all your online listings and assign someone on staff to repeat this exercise every 3–6 months.
3. Become an active participant in the rating and review process.
4. Set up Google and Yahoo! alerts for your name and clinic names, including obvious misspelled versions to monitor the web for unflattering posts and mentions.
5. Be proactive about engaging with patients to encourage them to post reviews on the sites that matter to your practice.

6. Take good care of patients and resolve conflicts early.
7. If or when they arise, try to bury negative comments with positive content so that these posts are not the first thing that comes up.

Updating Online Listings

Most rating and review sites allow you to claim your information and make updates. Hunt down every listing that you can. You want all the information about your practice to be as accurate and up to date as possible. Whenever possible, add hyperlinks to your website and social pages. Some sites require the physician to approve any changes and may even ask for your license number to verify your identity.

Having accurate listings does several important things for your clinic. It helps improve your website's ranking on search engines and increases the prominence of your placement in online searches. It also allows you to monitor what is being said about your practice so that you can respond or mitigate any negative comments.

The process of owning your listings will take some work in the beginning, but it will be worth it when your online reputation improves and new patients contact you for an appointment.

ONLINE REPUTATION CHECKLIST

1. Assign a staff member to manage the process and work with your web team for external support as needed.
2. List all the relevant sites and platforms that apply to your clinic.
3. Conduct a Google search at specific intervals using your name, the names of all the practitioners in your clinic, and the clinic's name.
4. Return to each site periodically after submitting updates to make sure that your changes have been made.
5. Set a regular date on your calendar to check back for new reviews and ratings (monthly or biweekly).
6. Look into directories, medical societies, and patient communities to make sure you have a listing in relevant platforms and that it is up to date.

ONLINE RATINGS CHEAT SHEET

Date	Site	Link	Information Listed	Reviews	Rating (stars)	Action
	Facebook					
	Google					
	Yelp					
	TripAdvisor					
	RealSelf					
	Healthgrades					

Another tactic is to look into patient communities that include listings of clinics and practitioners who see patients for specific conditions. For example, if you are a dermatologist or specialize in skin treatments, you may look at listing your practice on local, regional, or national resources for patients with common skin-related conditions like acne, rosacea, hair loss, and psoriasis.

Ratings and Reviews

WENDYISM

Downplaying the impact of patient reviews has on aesthetic practices is akin to burying your head in the proverbial sand.

A decade or so ago, one unhappy patient might tell a few of his/her friends about his/her doctor or complain about a less than perfect experience. Today, one unhappy patient can literally broadcast his/her displeasure to all of his/her fans and followers in a matter of seconds, and that can spread like flesh-eating bacteria all over the planet. Those fans and followers can, in turn, share this displeasure with their own fans and followers, and the end result can be gut wrenching for the practitioner. Once that unhappy patient presses the send button, his or her message is out there, and it is virtually indelible. All it takes is one person to share it, and it can take on a life of its own.

In an online universe dominated by search engines, reviews are among the first things prospective patients will see when searching for information. They may be exposed to reviews even if they aren't looking for them, as these tend to pop up everywhere you go online. Practitioners who ignore patient reviews are doing so at their own peril. Those who think that this is just a phase and will go away soon, are sadly mistaken. Consumer reviews are here to stay for every service and product, and will only get more important in the future. Your current and future patients are online reading what others have to say about you. The challenge is that a small number of people may be influencing what others think of you. To stay vigilant, you must listen to what people are saying about you and be a part of this conversation. You also need to encourage your happy patients to post reviews in an ethical way by avoiding any smell of incentives or impropriety.

Practitioners are understandably nervous about the impact of negative reviews. A few negative or not glowing reviews will not cause your clinic to shut down. However, even occasional reviews of 1, 2 and 3 stars can greatly impact your overall ratings. Clearly you need to aim for 4s and 5s continuously on the most relevant platforms to your practice.

Consumers are getting wiser to the process of reviews as well, and are much more likely to check out multiple sites to learn about a practitioner or clinic they are considering. Thus, having a good profile and ranking on one site may not overcome a less stellar rating on an other site. In many cases, 1 star reviews that begin with the ubiquitous ("If I could give this doctor zero stars, I would have ...) are often dismissed as a patient holding a grudge or fake. However, 2s and 3s definitely count among prospective patients and they read on to form an indelible impression.

REALSELF SURVEY RESULTS ON RATINGS AND REVIEWS

- In a RealSelf survey: 60% of RealSelf consumers said that finding the right doctor is the number one challenge
- 86% of consumers on RealSelf would not choose a doctor without a review
- In a RealSelf survey: 52% (the top answer) of RealSelf consumers said that they choose what doctor(s) to contact based on reviews
- In a RealSelf survey: 75% of RealSelf consumers said that they would be more likely to contact a doctor with 50 reviews and an average rating of 4.5 (out of 5 stars) vs a doctor with 10 reviews, who had an average rating of 5 (out of 5 stars)
- When (after consulting multiple doctors) a decision is made to select a doctor:
  - 29% of respondents said that comfort and trust was most important.
  - 22% said that reviews were the second more important thing in choosing a doctor.

Source: RealSelf Survey 2016, REALSELF.COM

Reputation Management Strategies

WENDYISM

Keep in mind that once you have a digital imprint online, it is almost impossible to remove.

If patient growth is a primary objective for your practice, and it should be, managing online reviews and ratings requires attention. Having accurate listings, engaging in the online conversation about your practice, building your online presence, and increasing reviews may be some of the most important things your practice can do to protect your reputation.

Physician management of negative online content can take many forms. Some approaches help distill an unflattering post, while others can backfire and escalate a situation. The last thing you want to do is to stimulate one comment and have it spread into a chain of like-minded comments.

Assign a staff member to watch what is being posted on all relevant sites and social networking platforms. Using an external monitoring service can also help alert you to any new developments, such as reposts of negative content and any derivative attacks that appear in response, so you can be proactive. As you check regularly on the review sites for new postings, be careful not to respond in a way that acknowledges a doctor-patient relationship.

Consumers are skeptical of reviews and look for red flags. You can make it worse by engaging with them in a public forum. If you feel compelled to reply, proceed with caution as a professional. Anyone who is reading these reviews is judging whether you are the kind of doctor they want to go to. Do not take risks online for all the world to see.

If you think a response is needed, it should be very straightforward, like "Thank you for expressing your concerns. Please be so kind as to contact our office so we can discuss this with you further. Patient satisfaction is our number one goal." Rather than the practitioner responding, it is wise to have a staff member be the point person. For less than four- or five-star reviews, try to take the conversation offline. Showing your willingness to be responsive can be almost as powerful as a positive review. In this way, you have demonstrated that you stand behind your reputation and pay attention to situations flagged in public forums. You can then privately try to resolve the conflict, assuming that the post is actually a real patient with a valid issue.

Common complaints on rating sites often center on long waiting times, a rushed staff, the doctor did not spend enough time, the feeling that the practice was too busy, and the ubiquitous bedside manner. You could try to distill the commentary about long waits and short visits with a statement, such as, "We are among only a few aesthetic practices in the area, and we pride ourselves on providing quality care to all of our patients." Do not be defensive, which can be misconstrued as arrogance.

There is always a risk of negative reviews appearing, so devise a strategy for how to respond to these critiques. It is important to listen to your patients and help resolve any negative experiences they may have had with you. When a negative comment is received, respond quickly to meet it head on. It may feel like an attack against you personally and/or your clinic. Take a deep breath before you address it. First assess the nature of the comment and respond only in a constructive way, if at all. Responding quickly is important, but it is equally wise to never respond in the heat of the moment when you are angry. Look at the situation from your perspective and that of the customer to give a balanced response.

Assign a staff member to monitor all of your social media sites to note any negative posts that were not posted by an actual patient. If you are the victim of a fake review or bogus anonymous comment, and this happens often, try to take the conversation offline and address it head on. On Facebook at least, you can delete the comment, ban the user from posting again, and report it as spam or inappropriate content.

Getting Posts Taken Down

Website hosts have significant latitude to keep or pull a thread. There are certain circumstances in which they are more likely to do so. Read the Terms of Service on the site very carefully. If the poster has violated the terms even slightly, you may have recourse to get the post removed. For example, Yelp's terms of service state that you must be a customer to post a comment, so this would be a clear violation and you might have some recourse, although nothing is guaranteed.

If you can prove that a post is fake—for example, a writer is complaining about a procedure that your clinic does not offer and you have evidence to substantiate that. If the post is just an opinion, you may be stuck. If the poster is stating something as fact that can be perceived as defamatory to your reputation, you may have a case to get the post taken down. But do not hold your breath. It is very hard to make a valid case to get posts taken down, and rather than spin your wheels and spend good money trying, I would urge you to invest that energy in doing everything you can to encourage five-star reviews from every patient.

Strategies for Generating Five-Star Reviews

A satisfied customer is the best business strategy of all.

Michael LeBoeuf

The best way to avoid negativity is to not create any reason for it in the first place. But this is nearly impossible anymore. The next best way to counter negative ratings is to make sure they are buried under a slew of positive ratings from real satisfied patients who are your advocates.

So, how do you get patients to post good reviews? Sometimes you have to ask them. It is much easier for staff to ask than the doctor. When a patient compliments the result, office, or staff, it is very easy for the staff to say to the patient, "You will make our day if you give us a positive review." There is no shame in doing that. In fact, it has become common practice among all service businesses, including hotels, restaurants, salons, airlines, and even Uber and eBay. The practitioner can do the same, if he or she has the kind of relationship with the patient that feels comfortable. Just asking a patient may not be enough as the thought passes out of his or her mind immediately after leaving your office. Giving the patient a card with various rating sites may be a good reminder. Having patients write reviews while they are in your office will not work because they will come from the same ISP address and will not be considered legitimate.

Start the process from the initial consultation when the patients are sitting in the waiting room. Use patient satisfaction surveys to show patients that you value their opinion, and get them to participate.

Encouraging patients to post good reviews about your practice is a constant battle, but the rewards will pay off. Be consistent. Do all you can, every day, to garner positive ratings. If you don't, you will fall into the rut of getting a negative rating and then suddenly scrambling for some good reviews, which will be very apparent when someone looks at the site.

Honest doctors may admit that the threat of negative reviews has made them just a little more caring and humble as they know that there are more consequences to bad behavior than in the past. There is that little voice inside your head that keeps telling you to just be nice and smile more. Maybe that is not such a bad thing after all. Everyone will get some negative reviews—some unwarranted, yet some deserved. No one likes it. When it happens, first look in the mirror and ask, "Hey, is there some truth in this critique?" Use this as an opportunity to improve how you do things, rather than just getting your back up and acting defensively. If there is a flaw in your system, address it and deal with it directly. If your bedside manner is the main issue, do a little soul searching.

WENDYISM

Let's face it. If you are consistently getting three stars or less, there may be a few things that demand your immediate attention.

When you find content that addresses a genuine shortcoming in your practice, use it as an opportunity to improve. Develop an approach that instills trust and confidence with each patient visit. If you have to rush to get through a busy day of patients, apologize to anyone who has been kept waiting and explain why. Get the staff involved in answering questions and moving patients through more quickly. Make an extra effort to avoid scheduling mishaps and billing snafus that are sure to cause patients to be irate. Another patient pet peeve is promising to do something and letting it slip through the cracks—such as calling back, contacting their insurance company, sending a receipt, making a copy of a chart, or calling in a prescription.

A collection of sincerely favorable reviews by real patients will outweigh a few negative ones, so being vigilant about fostering goodwill with patients is even more critical now. Persuade patients to write good reviews about your practice by showing that it matters to you. Include positive reviews on your website and brochures and feature them throughout your social media platforms. Post a sign at the reception desk stating that you value patient feedback by any means, including in person, by phone or e-mail, or via online forums.

Your ongoing mission is to create a large body of positive content to outweigh any negative posts that may arise—and they will.

Avoiding Legal Action

When you go online, you leave electronic footprints almost everywhere you go. So, if you want to track down someone who has posted about you, you may be able to get their personal information if they gave an ISP or message board when they signed up (name, address, phone number, e-mail, etc.). Some sites might only have required an e-mail address to register. In this case, a subpoena to the ISP that hosts that address will be necessary to obtain the individual's true identity. But it is not that simple. Ask yourself if doing an exhaustive search is really going to be worth your time and trouble. If you are successful in finding out who the individuals may be, you will not have much recourse to go after them.

Physicians have tried to file lawsuits against patients or doctor rating sites over negative reviews, but they usually lose. It is better to address grievances and complaints by encouraging the patient to come back to the clinic, rather than tackling it online, which may escalate. It is ill advised to allow a bad review.

12 KEY RATINGS AND REVIEW SITES TO MONITOR
- RealSelf
- Google
- Facebook
- Yelp
- TripAdvisor
- Healthgrades
- RateMDs
- Vitals
- Healthcare Reviews
- Doctoralia
- TopDoctors
- WhatClinic

Dealing with Negative Posts and Tweets

Negative comments or bogus posts are always a possibility on social media. These can be from random strangers, spammers, and competitive web marketing companies. In some cases, unfortunately, off-color comments may be from actual patients. The fear of negative comments can be a tremendous deterrent for some practitioners to become active in online forums.

The good news, however, is that you have the ability to control who posts on your wall, anything can be removed, and the user can be blocked and reported to Facebook. However, I would urge you to think twice before you do that unless it is abusive or fake. If the post is a comment about pricing or something else benign, you may want to address it—without acknowledging a doctor-patient relationship. When you get rid of it, you just make someone mad. If you delete it on Facebook, which is the only platform you can really do that on easily, the same person who may now be even more annoyed with you, can post it on Yelp, or create a new Facebook account and post it again on Facebook. You may not actually be putting the fire out. Try to take the matter offline and urge the poster to contact the clinic by using Facebook Messenger, e-mail, or phone. This also shows your fans that the clinic is interested in patient care.

On Twitter you have no control at all, so if you see a negative tweet, it is generally best to leave it alone. The risk of responding may be worse than leaving it because Twitter is real time, and if you do not respond in 3 minutes, it is out there. You can try to send a direct message to the Twitter user, which is private, to take it offline.

It is possible to convert unhappy customers to brand advocates if complaints are handled swiftly and proficiently. Patients want to know that you care about them and that they are being heard.

Patient Privacy Considerations

Practitioners must keep all patient details anonymous at all times. Get educated on rules and regulations your membership organizations and local health authorities may have regarding social media use, as these can vary widely.

Even now, many cosmetic patients do not want to receive mail, phone calls, e-mails, or other communications that are identified as coming from an aesthetic clinic. In the interest of patient confidentiality, the clinic staff should specifically ask every patient how they wish to be contacted by the clinic; for example, home, mobile, office phone, e-mail, or via postal mail. Some may not want to be contacted at all, and that request should be honored.

If you are going to use any patients' photos—even if the face is not showing or the eyes are blacked out—written consent is mandatory. The same goes for patient videos or any photos of patients who may have attended a seminar in your clinic. Explain to patients exactly what the consent they are signing covers in order to avoid misunderstandings. Make it clear if their photographs and videos will be used for internal clinic training, external teaching at meetings and conferences, on websites, and on which social media platforms.

DOCTOR'S ORDERS

- Refrain from friending or reaching out to past or current patients on social media.
- Keep your business accounts (which users may "like" and follow without breaching the practitioner-patient relationship) and personal accounts separate to avoid confusion.
- If someone reaches out to you through electronic means who is not a patient, use your best judgment about engaging, and redirect that person to call or schedule a consultation at your clinic to answer any questions he or she may have.
- Let the patient do the engaging, such as liking your professional business page.
- If a patient tries to friend the practitioner on his or her personal Facebook profile, common practice is not to accept the friend request.
- Never acknowledge, whether directly or indirectly, any doctor-patient relationship in an online forum.
- Posting anything about specific cases, revealing any patient information, or making comments that could be misconstrued as a breach are a no-go.
- Refrain from offering medical advice or suggesting anything that would require a consultation with a practitioner first.

A practitioner's personal behavior as well as his or her clinic's actions in online forums carry some risk. Stay abreast of general professional guidelines for social media that are constantly under evaluation. To protect your license and reputation, check with your malpractice insurance carrier. This is an evolving area, and the law has not kept up with the rapid speed at which this space is moving.

Anyone you assign to post or engage on social media for your clinic should be well versed in the guidelines that apply to your clinic and specialty. That includes staff, external consultants, public relations team, webmaster, or marketing agency. Everyone needs to be on the same page to preserve the boundaries of the doctor-patient relationship when interacting with patients online and ensure that patient privacy and confidentiality are strictly maintained.

In general, you should adhere to the same principles of professionalism online as offline. Compliance with patient privacy regulations is critical, and practitioners must remember to keep all patient details anonymous. If you are unclear on the best guidelines for navigating these uncharted waters, seek legal advice. The consequences can be huge.

Stay Calm and Carry On

In reality, it is impossible to have 100% happy patients despite your best efforts. Regrettably, ratings sites and social media platforms have become the obvious places for patients and customers to vent and air their grievances. They are the first port of call for spite-based attacks on your professional reputation, and unfortunately, some patients use these platforms as a weapon.

No matter how good you are as a practitioner, you are bound to get some snide remarks about your fees and complaints about your approach or attitude at some point. It is almost impossible not to, especially if you have a busy practice. The more patients you treat, the higher the odds are of having some unhappy campers in the bunch.

It can be difficult to stay calm when you read what people are writing about you online. The worst thing you can do is to react in a defensive or aggressive manner. Try to stay rational, and reasonable, even when the patient is completely unreasonable. Whenever possible, keep emotions out of it. As a licensed healthcare professional, you do not share the privilege of overreacting with your patients.

Communicating with Patients Online

Are Your Messages to Patients Encrypted?

If you have to ask yourself this question, they probably aren't. Instant messaging via texts or SMS, is a popular and handy method of communication. Although it is perfectly fine for talking to your family and friends, it can pose potential risks for practitioners because this type of correspondence is not secure and can easily be intercepted by others. The same is true for FaceTime® and SKYPE® and Facebook Messenger.

This is especially challenging when it comes to communicating directly with patients or with other healthcare providers directly about patients. Your data and medical records may be compromised. New ways of communicating in cyberspace are way ahead of regulations and continue to fall behind. The traditional ways of making, confirming, changing appointments, asking questions, checking in pre- and post-procedures by mail and phone are no longer efficient methods.

Patients depend on mobile devices 24/7, so it is natural to want to hear from dermatologists and cosmetic surgeons via texting, especially for routine communications such as appointment reminders and prescription renewals. This method of interaction enables patients to connect with their doctors in a way they feel most comfortable, which in turn can help to enhance the doctor–patient relationship. It may also help to promote increased loyalty to the practice, and cut down on cancellations and no-shows.

However for messaging to be secure, it is essential that these communications must be encrypted before they ever get transferred from your device. Basically, encrypted messages can only be read by the intended recipient. Even if your message gets intercepted during the exchange, it is still safe and protected from spying eyes.

Therefore, what is a practitioner supposed to do? Download an app or subscribe to a platform that offers services to encrypt your data before you send it through normal unsafe channels. Search for "secure messaging solutions" to find out more about the options currently available for IOS and Android devices.

6

The Secret Sauce of Content Marketing

The future of publishing is about having connections to readers and the knowledge of what those readers want.

Seth Godin

The art of creating great content that connects with readers is more of a science.

There are certain elements that, if you infuse them into your content, will make it more relatable and impactful for your readers. Here are some tried-and-true tips for creating content that resonates with your target audiences and will (hopefully) keep them following, liking, and sharing your content.

Better Blogging

A blog, or web log, is essentially an online shared journal that gets frequently updated with brief bursts of content about your topics of choice. Blogging is a viable platform for promoting your clinic and an important way to get your clinic moving up on search rankings. Blogging allows you to do so much more than just share news and promote events. You can use a blog to boost your credibility, create a personal connection with your audience, and answer questions and queries.

Blogging is not all about controlling the dialogue—it is an organic evolution of a conversation. Many physicians incorporate a blog as a special subsection of their websites, while others create a separate domain name for their blog, such as drsmithsblog.com.

Unlike Twitter that requires status updates to be made throughout the day to be meaningful, or a Facebook page that demands at least one post daily, blogging is a less time-intensive undertaking. You may choose to blog once a week, or preferably more, and the frequency of posting can vary. If you like writing and are willing to invest the time and effort to think of interesting topics for your posts, blogging can actually be an enjoyable pursuit. But if blogging is just going to become another thing on your "to-do" list, delegating it to a staff member or enlisting the services of a professional beauty or health writer is the best way to maintain a blog. Another good way to add content to your blog is to provide updated headlines and news articles from other sites that are of interest to your followers. These posts may include commentaries and recommendations compiled by the practitioner or clinic to make the content uniquely your own.

Allowing comments can enable discussion on your site and turn it into an interactive social place for people to visit. It can also increase social media optimization. You can set up the blog so that all comments require approval to go live to avoid spammers or inappropriate posts.

Staying on Message

The clutter of content online means people actually appreciate brevity and a targeted message that speaks directly to them. Finding the ideal online voice for your clinic and sticking with it can be tricky, especially if you are not creating the content yourself.

Once you have found your voice, the next step is to identify the buckets of content that your fans and followers relate to most, and to continue to create new and unique variations on those key themes. An integrated social media marketing plan starting with a blog is a critical element of success.

Maintaining a professional image and tone online is essential. Resist the temptation to come across as flippant or overly self-promotional, which can backfire on your reputation with patients. As a healthcare practitioner, you should strive to be taken seriously and offer reasonable opinions and solid advice that attract real patients to come in for consultation and have treatments in your practice.

Getting Started

Creating a blog is actually a relatively affordable and simple process. The real obstacle is finding the time to maintain a blog by developing content that is relevant to your readers.

BLOG PLATFORMS

Platform	Details
WordPress	Premium fully customizable blog and website platform—universally most used
Blogger	Free blogging platform
Squarespace	Do-it-yourself (DIY) website, blog, shop builder with customizable templates, 24/7 support
Wix	DIY website builder with customizable templates
Weebly	DIY website builder with customizable templates
Ghost	Free open-source publishing platform
Joomla!	Mobile-ready and user-friendly website builder

The most popular blog program is WordPress, which looks more professional than other platforms and is relatively easy to use. Ideally, a professional blog should be set up by a programmer who can install the requisite widgets and plug-ins to make your blog more interactive. You will need help to properly install widgets and other useful applications that can be embedded into your blog. Widgets can be used to greatly enhance your blog productivity. Widgets are programs that display information or create efficient ways to help readers interact with your blog. Widgets may include icons, pull-down menus, buttons, selection boxes, scroll bars, windows, links, toggle buttons, and many other technical formats for displaying information and allowing readers to interact. Due to the highly technical nature of widgets, they are best managed by a programmer.

I would only recommend using the low-tech do-it-yourself (DIY) platforms if you are on a tight budget and are just starting out. These sites may look good, but they are harder to work with from a technical perspective. It is well worth investing in a quality, professionally designed and programmed website and blog for your clinic that can be updated regularly to stay on top of the trends.

WENDYISM

I do not inject my own Botox, so why would a highly trained aesthetic practitioner want to design his or her own website or blog? Stick to what you know.

Integrate a Blog with Your Website

Ideally a blog should have the same look and feel as your clinic website. It can either be set up to live within your site or under a separate domain name to increase search engine rank. Most practices will choose the former. You may wish to host your blog within your primary domain (e.g., wendylewisco .com/blog or blog.wendylewisco.com) instead of hosting your blog externally (e.g., skinclinic.wordpress.

com). Try not to cannibalize search engine optimization (SEO) authority by having two domains compete against each other. Every time you start a new domain name, you need to set aside a budget for SEO and Pay-Per-Click (PPC) to get found.

The challenge for practitioners is finding the time to blog and then deciding what to blog about. One of the best ways to add engaging and meaningful content to your blog is to curate interesting content that is already posted on medical websites and Facebook pages. You can then add your own spin to make it uniquely yours. Find good content by searching on social media platforms, medical blogs, medical portals, and health and beauty publications. Set Google alerts for key categories and topics, such as cosmetics, laser resurfacing, dermatologic surgery, skin cancer, cosmetic surgery, sun protection, acne treatments, skin care, and so on.

A blog can be a useful tool for getting your message across, educating consumers and media, keeping your patients informed of developments or newsworthy items, and providing carefully restrained venting on selected topics. At least one mission of blogging should be to convert traffic to readers, subscribers, and followers who are interested in what you have to say. You may also use your blog to elicit feedback or input from patients and followers, like a focus group or survey.

To help with search engine visibility, posts should be optimized by including keywords in the text, such as "laser resurfacing Sydney," while keeping it readable. Blog posts can usually be scheduled in advance, and frequency should be at least once weekly to keep the momentum going.

Get up to speed on the Google friendly language needed to optimize your blog posts for maximum marketing effect. You can channel your creative juices to produce a steady flow of organized blog posts, but like Twitter, Facebook, texting, and other platforms of modern communication, blogging has a language of its own. It may seem that Google, Yahoo!, and Bing dictate what is a good blog; however, the best blogs contain a balance of good writing, humor, compassion, and personality, as well as hidden search terms and strategically placed links.

If your posts are all about search engine optimization (SEO), you may achieve a higher search engine ranking, but you may not develop a following of readers who actually pay attention to your content. By using key phrases, keywords, and search terms to optimize your blog content, you can bring more readers to you. However, it will impose restraints on your writing style and add an extra layer to the process.

To optimize the titles of blog posts directly for the search engines, include a keyword in your title, preferably near the beginning. But do not stop there; optimizing titles for readers is also important. Titles should attract the readers' attention and let them know what your post is all about and how they will benefit from reading it.

Do not overuse keywords; stick with a main keyword in the introductory paragraph and use another keyword at the end of the post. The rest of the content should be readable and make sense. If you load up your blog posts with "Cheshire Cosmetic Clinic" or "Top Revision Rhinoplasty Surgeon," you have lost the plot. Search engines are wise to this methodology, and they can even identify synonyms faster than you can say "ROGET." Consumers find it monotonous, and you may end up with a high bounce rate. If your plan is to get more likes and shares, the content has to say something worthwhile and be presented in an engaging way.

Content should be readable and interesting to resonate with your target audience, educate and inform, and ring true to your brand. Blogs written in the practitioner's voice need to sound authentic. Consider adding a disclaimer to your blog, as you should have on your website footer, specifying that "Content contained herein is not a substitute for a consultation with a medical doctor and should not be considered medical advice." If you are unclear on the appropriate language to use, contact your lawyer or malpractice carrier for guidance to limit potential liability.

In some cases, creating a blog under a new domain name that lives on its own can offer more marketing muscle than merely adding a blog to your landing page. Be careful about spreading your SEO/PPC budget too thin by having to market an additional URLs. For maximum effectiveness, blog content should also be leveraged on your Facebook page, Twitter, and all other social channels you are active on. Blog content can also be repurposed in e-mail blasts and newsletters for maximum effect. Choose to create evergreen or generic blog content that does not get outdated, so you can get more out of your effort.

Blog Structure

There are several key elements that should be built into every blog post, and they all play an important role in getting the most mileage for your blog. It is advisable not to date blog posts. Readers are more likely to only go to the most recent posts and may tend to spend less time on your blog if they think the posts are too old.

WENDYISM

Use the right format for the right type of content to reach the right audience.

A blog is better suited to short-form content, whereas an e-book will have a more captive audience, interested in scrolling through more pages and charts, because someone had to fill out a form with personal information to redeem it. If you are debating whether to create a video blog post or text, determine the content format that will help you get your message across in the clearest way, and the way your audience will enjoy consuming it best.

Make it easy for readers to learn more about your clinic, staff, products, and services by including navigation to primary business pages. The goal is to encourage them to stay and read more. Encourage readers to browse through all of the available content by grouping by topic such as Skincare, Acne Treatments, Fat Reduction, Hair Restoration, and also by content type (such as video, infographic, statistics, or survey).

The average reader has a pretty short attention span when it comes to reading content online. Try to make your posts scannable because most online readers will not read every word. Their eyes go to certain words and phrases first so they can get the gist of what you are writing about before they decide to devote any more time to it.

Long posts created purely for the sake of extra words are not really effective. Short blurbs that do not say enough are also not so interesting to readers or Google. If the post is too long, chances are visitors will not read to the end. Try to write posts of the length that it takes you to communicate what you want to say. Mixing long, medium, and short posts is fine; not every post has to be the same word count. If you add compelling visuals and links, you can reduce the word count. Shorter posts allow you to write more posts, which is preferable for generating readership with RSS and on search engines.

RSS FEED

RSS (Rich Site Summary) is a format for delivering regularly changing web content. News sites, blogs, and other online publishers syndicate their content as an RSS feed online. **Whatisrss.com**

A good guideline is to make your blog posts no more than 600 words and no less than 300 words. The type of post you are writing will determine the right length. For example, if you are writing about your opinion on a new procedure, you may write more than if you are relating the details of a news item where you will link to the full story so the reader can find out more. If you have a lot to say on a particular topic, splitting a long post into a series of shorter posts can be a great way to keep readers coming back. They can read Part 1 and return to read Part 2 at a future date.

Your first paragraph is both an introductory and summary section; introduce the reader to the reason for your post. The body of the post should include links to social networking platforms. You can also let viewers skim your content by previewing posts in parts. Make the preview even more clickable by adding an image. Vary the posts on the blog to feature photos, videos, press clips, links, and graphics to make each post more interesting.

Entries should include share buttons so readers can recycle the content on their social media platforms. More is more for search engine visibility. If multiple people will be contributing to the blog, the options are to write every post yourself as the "authority" in the first person, or to craft posts in the third person or the "we" voice from the clinic as an entity. Each post can also be identified by the individual author, such as a clinic manager, aestheticians, and individual practitioners. The most practical way to go may be to outsource your blog to a professional health, beauty, or medical writer whom you can trust to get it right.

Choosing Categories

Blog categories allow you to organize your posts by topic and let your readers easily find the topics that are the most interesting to them. Whenever possible, use relevant keywords and popular brands name your categories. This allows readers to easily search for relevant posts.

10 BLOG POST CATEGORY EXAMPLES
- Anti-aging
- Laser resurfacing
- Facial fillers
- Fat grafting
- Lip enhancement
- Fat reduction
- Microdermabrasion
- Sun protection
- Skincare
- Botox

Keyword Tags

Put yourself in the mind of the reader when you choose keywords. For example, if your clinic specializes in nonsurgical antiaging treatments for women, start off with some basic categories that prospective patients might look for, such as "wrinkle reduction treatments," "wrinkle reducing injections," "nonsurgical facelift," or "skin rejuvenation." Expand your keyword list by including product or brand names that resonate with consumers, such as "Botox injections," "facial fillers," "skin tightening systems," or "lasers."

Include keywords in your post title, header tag, image text, copy, and meta-description. Each blog post can be associated with keywords. Choose keywords that are related to the topic and also use these keywords in the content.

Add a Meta-Description

A meta-description is a summary of your web page for search engines. Make sure your blog has one that includes keywords so that searchers will know what your blog is about. This area allows you to include a description of your post. Create the description by using some keywords, for example, "*Visit Liverpool Skin Clinic—Top Rated Clinic for Aesthetic Treatments in the North—If you are looking for the best therapies to reverse the signs of aging, book a consultation with our skin experts.*"

Title Tag

Instead of calling your blog "Skin Clinic's Blog," you can use keywords here as well. Since search engines put more emphasis on words closer to the left, name your blog's page title something that focuses on keywords first, then your company name, to gain authority for those keywords. The title tag area gives you some flexibility to be creative. Create post titles that are interesting and make the reader want to read more.

The Importance of Visuals

Search engines can read the file names of your photos. If you are using a photo or two in a post, use a keyword for the file name when you save it to your laptop. Name images strategically before uploading them to your post, and include alternative text in case your image does not show up for the user. If you are posting patient photos, make sure the patient's name has been removed and that you have a properly drafted and signed consent on file. Avoid making blog posts a wall of just text. Include at least one image to make your blog reader friendly and in the style of an online magazine. Video content is a useful element to engage readers, and search engines.

Internal Text Links

Within each blog post, you can include links to other content in your blog or on your website. Whether you are referencing your product, service, or a topic featured in another blog post, use keyword-rich anchor text to create the link. This gives search engines more information about the content of that page. Navigate to other content in your blog structure, and also link to relevant content within the post itself. Include internal links, to pages within your domain, with anchor text to help readers find more content and rank for keywords.

Calls to Action

Think about what you want readers to do when they are on your blog. Make sure every blog post includes at least one keyword and well-crafted call to action (CTA). These can be at the beginning or end of the post, sidebar, or links within the copy itself.

10 TRENDING BLOG TOPICS

- Erasing acne scars
- Early skin cancer detection saves lives
- Best fillers for lips and lines
- Back to school skincare regime
- New laser speeds up tattoo removal
- Sculpt your body without surgery
- Cheekbones are back!
- Summer bodies are made in winter
- Here comes the bride and she is glowing
- Get party ready for the holidays

At the core of every successful blog is great content. How you define "great" content will vary somewhat, but it should be content that is unique and relevant to the reader (for more information on calls to action, see Chapter 2).

Preferred Posting Practices

What happens when you post another entry to your blog? A few people may read or view it. Some may even post comments or share with a friend. Most blog posts will not gain much momentum unless someone is driving the marketing of your blog. Rather than viewing publishing a post as the end point, it is just the beginning.

Promoting blogs should be integrated into your overall online strategy to drive traffic and build brand awareness. Leverage every new post by reaching out to other bloggers. Having another blog or blogger recommend something you posted to their followers or people who trust them is a very powerful way to get the word out. However, getting other bloggers to link to your posts takes some effort. If you do not have an established profile or a preexisting relationship with the bloggers you are pitching, they may not respond.

Avoid pitching posts to other bloggers unless your blog has direct relevance to their readers. Only pitch your most interesting and unique posts that have a higher success rate of getting a link. Avoid suggesting links to purely self-promotional posts, which are most likely to be declined. Offer an angle to the blogger, such as what your post is about and why it might be relevant to their blog. Personalize your request with the name of the blogger and the blog to show that you have a specific interest and are not just casting a wide net. Ultimately, it will be up to the blogger to decide if your blog is relevant for him or her, and some may ask for a fee, which can be worth it if the traffic is substantial.

Try to get your blog included in other bloggers' blogrolls. A blogroll is a list of links, usually located on the sidebar, that the blogger enjoys and wants to share with his or her readers. This is often a reciprocal relationship. A blogger might use a blogroll to help promote their friends' blogs or offer readers a wider array of resources on a particular niche, such as beauty or skincare.

Promote yourself from within your blog by using automated and customized tools to drive traffic from your blog to social networks. There are a plethora of social widgets that can be installed by a programmer. Even if you opt for an automated tool as a time-saving measure, widgets work best if you diversify by adding your own personal tweets, linking to external content, and asking questions of readers. Foster community by engaging in a dialogue.

Think of your blog as a dynamic entity with a unique personality of its own. Linking back to your own blog keeps readers engaged and encourages them to explore more of your content. If you search by word or category, you can find a few posts in your archives that you can link back to a current post. Add a link to other content where you may have discussed similar topics as "related reading." Internal links also improve your search engine optimization.

If you keep your content visible, relevant, and unique, you can attract the right kind of positive attention that adds to your credibility as a trusted source of balanced information.

6 TIPS FOR BETTER BLOGGING

1. Engage readers with a catchy title to draw them in.
2. Ask the reader for a response to draw him or her in.
3. End every blog with a call to action (CTA).
4. Add a "Share This" plugin that allows you to automatically add social media sharing buttons on every post.
5. Add a search box on the sidebar so users can find exactly what they are looking for.
6. Encourage readers to follow your content by including a link to subscribe to your content via e-mail to help build your list and/or RSS feed.

Guest Blogging

Guest posting has become widely accepted method of adding links to be placed on websites, blogs, forums, and comments sections. Sites that accept free contributions usually do not have any standards at all. Strategic links back to clients' sites that get included in these articles are often painful to read due to the awkward language and optimization tactics. So, when you see a feature that repeats phrases like "Hamburg Laser Surgeon" or "Best Bodyshaping Boston" 10 times in one paragraph, it is a thinly disguised SEO exercise. Guest blogging purely for SEO purposes is frowned upon.

Public relations (PR) professionals often suggest writing and pitching "bylined articles." The key difference between a byline and a guest post is that a bylined article may provide relevant content that also serves the needs of the client by positioning him or her as an expert on a particular topic.

Submitting articles with your byline for publication on select websites can be a highly effective strategy to increase traffic to your site, if you have a hyperlink included in the copy.

Benefits of e-Books

An e-book is essentially a booklet created in a downloadable digital format that is usually offered at no charge to interested readers. Choose a theme that is a hot topic generate buzz for your brand. Think of magazine articles that patients would want to read, such as "A New Way to Lift a Sagging Neck—No Surgery Required" or "Freeze Your Mummy Tummy in Your Lunch Hour." Include visuals that tell the story to break up text. Because these are not designed to be printed, you can create e-books as short or long as you like. From 4 to 12 pages is a good range to work with.

An e-book can be used as a hook to build your e-mail list. Marketing an e-book is straightforward and cost effective. Your Facebook page is the perfect platform to start with. You can offer a free e-book from your page in return for fans filling out a simple form to capture their name, e-mail, and some demographic information.

To attract followers who will want to read your e-book, a Facebook ad campaign is highly recommended. Give people some copy to entice them to download it and a reason they will want to read it. Promoting an e-book on social media is a cost-effective way to reach a very targeted audience.

To make sure your e-book delivers real value, offer useful tips and insider information. Do not just regurgitate copy that is already available on your site or blog or make it a marketing pitch. Keep it fresh with an upbeat tone that is readable and lively, yet informative and visually appealing. It is preferable to enlist the services of a professional writer to work with you for these projects who can keep the tone and voice consistent with your brand. If your sign-ups do not like the e-book, they will lose interest in your clinic and services and will not convert, so the effort will be futile.

8 GREAT E-BOOK THEMES

1. Take 10 Years Off Your Face In 10 Minutes
2. The New Way to Restore Your Hairline Without Scars
3. Get Your Confidence Back With Women's Laser Therapy
4. Breakthrough Skincare To Turn Back the Clock
5. Safer Breast Implants
6. How To Get A Sexy Summer Body
7. New Year, New (insert body part here)
8. Six Steps to a Younger You

Another popular way to get your views and key messages across on popular topics is to create your own podcast. A podcast is essentially like an audio blog post that subscribers can download the listen to on their smartphones.

7

Getting Social Media Savvy

I come from a culture where the pub is the centre of the community. The pub is the Internet. It's where information is gathered, collated and addressed.

Rhys Ifans

Social media has ignited at a rapid pace and new platforms are emerging on a daily basis, and the value it can bring to aesthetic clinics is also on the rise. It has undoubtedly transformed how all businesses communicate directly and openly with customers, and has revolutionized how we receive and share news and information.

Aesthetic practitioners have to be ready to meet the demands of mastering social media to engage with existing patients and increase visibility with prospective patients. Having a Facebook page for your clinic allows you to promote your business, interact with existing and potential clients, and create positive relationships. You will be able to talk about the services you offer, products you sell, and procedures you perform. But Facebook is just the place to begin. There are many additional platforms that offer new opportunities for clinics to build their brand.

The challenge is finding the time to do it all, as well as learning how to stand out and getting your message across effectively and with the right tone. Whether you are just starting on a social media marketing strategy, designing a new campaign, or trying to figure out if Snapchat makes sense, get up to speed on the most relevant platforms, who uses them, why, and how.

MVPs (MOST VALUABLE PLATFORMS)

Platform	Active Monthly Users
FB—Facebook	2 billion
TW—Twitter	328 million
IG—Instagram	700 million
LI—LinkedIn	400 million
SC—Snapchat	301 million
G+—Google+	540 million
YT—YouTube	1.5 billion
Pinterest	200 million

Source: https://www.thesocialmediahat.com/active-users (as of July 15, 2017).

Note that social media metrics change constantly and are calculated differently by various outlets, so it is hard to get exact numbers for unique monthly visitors or active users at any given time. Factor in the hordes of fake accounts and users that get booted off daily, and the numbers may seem a bit inflated.

Social media platforms have enabled physicians to be more visible to patients in exciting ways. They provide an ideal venue for humor and other forms of creative content. If you create quality content, your fans will come back for more. The content that excites your fans is what gets shared, forwarded, and linked to from other sites. This is what keeps people reading and drives conversions.

Undoubtedly, most successful clinics are already heavily invested online and have developed a robust web presence over time. Social media now plays a vital role in marketing for an aesthetic practice. But this new way of marketing is constantly changing, which can be overwhelming, confusing, and downright frustrating for the novice and the veteran alike. It takes time and effort to build up engagement and reach on social platforms, and a strategic plan must consider the clinic's brand position. A haphazard approach to social media is sure to fail.

Two-Way Dialogue

WENDYISM

There is no golden rule book for doing social right—except that it takes a village.

With the staggering numbers, it is getting harder for aesthetic practices to stand out in the digital world. It takes a double dose of ingenuity and a creative mind-set to build a community and keep them engaged. Social media users are a fickle bunch. They are easily distracted by the next new thing and have the ability to quickly screen out anything that does not catch their interest. If your campaign fails to entice and encourage participation, social media users can be brutal. If you miss the mark, they are not so shy about telling you so. As aesthetic practitioners know all too well, happy, satisfied customers are less likely to go public, say thank you, or write glowing reviews and endorsements. Disgruntled patients tend to be more vocal, proactive, often tell you what they do not like, and expect an immediate response.

True or False? Social media is only important during normal business hours.

False: Social media is a 24/7, 365 days/year thing. People will be posting on social networks on their mobile devices at any time during the day or night. Each platform is also different in terms of peak times for interactions. Just because your clinic is closed on Sunday does not mean people are not on Facebook on Sundays. National holidays offer great opportunities to post because there is so much more you can say.

Someone must be minding the store, responding to posts and queries, creating interesting content, and engaging with fans and followers 24/7. You should aim to respond to every reasonable comment as quickly as possible, and deal with negative posts head on.

An hour a day when the receptionist is not busy is not enough to maintain your brand on social media. The clinic receptionist should be answering the phones promptly and dealing with patients efficiently, without the distraction of liking pages and retweeting posts.

Social media has changed the nature of interactions among consumers and brands in four key ways:

1. **User-generated content**
2. **Building community**
3. **Real-time conversation**
4. **Two-way dialogue**

Social media platforms always seem like they were designed by and developed by younger age groups—teens, collegiates, and millennials. Most social networks start with that audience as its core demographic since they are the early adopters. As each network starts to catch on, the audience invariably expands. Look at how Facebook started as a network built exclusively for college students. Today, college students have moved away from Facebook, partially because their parents are all over it so it lost its hipness. Now even grandmas are using Facebook to keep in touch and share family photos.

Instagram and Snapchat are among the fastest growing platforms. They are not quite Facebook yet in terms of sheer numbers, but they are no longer niche social networks that you can ignore. Social media has become increasingly diversified, as content is more engaging and visual. The key is to choose the platforms best suited to your target audience. It has become increasingly more difficult to differentiate yourself on platforms with hundreds of millions or billions of users, and an ad strategy has become mandatory to get seen.

While having a lot of likes on Facebook is certainly important, actual engagement, human interaction, and two-way conversions remain the overriding goals of social media. Sustainable growth requires clever storytelling, authentic branding, user-generated campaigns, and quality content. You need to be present where your target audience is going, and be an early adopter on those key channels.

Let your audience know where they can find you so they do not miss out on your posts. Add social buttons and usernames on all your marketing materials, including your website, blog, all other social media channels, e-blasts, business cards, newsletters, and all consumer-facing practice materials. Whenever possible, secure the same username throughout all social media channels for consistency and to make it easier for patients to find you.

It is better to be on your platforms of choice in frequent bursts than to put in an hour or two randomly throughout the week. Key time savers include the ability to preschedule updates and tools that can update multiple platforms at once. Scheduling aids have transformed social media posting and tracking. For example, Facebook has a built-in scheduler on business pages. Hootsuite and others subscription-based platforms enable scheduling for multiple social channels from a single dashboard (see Chart of Social Media Management Tools on pages 59, 70).

Be careful not to utilize terminology that is specific to only one or two social networks. It can be confusing to post a status update on Facebook that uses hashtags that are specific to Twitter and Instagram. If you are posting across networks, make sure your message works for all of them by changing the format and style to match the users.

Learn which platforms are most relevant for your marketing goals, and how to maximize performance on those key platforms to reap the greatest rewards. Link back to your website by posting your URL on Twitter, Facebook, and so on, to drive people back to your website so that your activities are not just purely conversational. When you are tweeting, Facebooking, or blogging, you can continually send people back to your to capture their e-mail addresses. Social media platforms may come and go and waver in popularity, but your e-mail lists are marketing gold.

Break down social media into platforms that are mandatory and those that are optional, based on the clinic's primary and secondary target audiences, goals, budget, and manpower. You do not have to use every social media platform, but at least set up a profile on the best of or at least reserve your clinic name. Use the same username across all or most of them for consistency and clarity. So the process is less overwhelming, implement one platform at a time, and then focus on those that have the highest return for your practice. Invest the most time and money on the sites the majority of your patients are most active on.

Technically, you should not be using the same content in the same way for every social platform. Consider which platform your post is the best fit for, and change the way it is used on other platforms. For example, if you are hosting a patient seminar, think about whether it would work better for Twitter or is it Snapchat worthy? Is just posting a group photo on Instagram enough? Or should you put it on Facebook and Twitter to generate the most views. You cannot just tweet and post about how great you are every day, or your audience will stop paying attention. This is not what social media is all about. It is about a dialogue and sharing. The secret is to make it interactive, like asking a question or crowdsourcing.

Engagement Strategies

Social media has redefined the rules for how business is done and, thus, how successful clinics are run. This sea change has had sweeping effects on medical aesthetics. For example, the traditional, one-way ad campaign has evolved into a more personal and dynamic two-way dialogue. This allows clinics to really connect and engage with their customers.

Start by figuring out the platforms that your patients are on, and expand from there. Looking at social media becomes overwhelming, so we want to dissect it and bring it to a level that you are comfortable with and that is manageable in-house.

Know, Like, Trust

Building trust with your customers is like dating. The courtship phase does not happen overnight. It takes time, powers of persuasion, and a healthy dose of sensitivity.

Social media can help to increase the "know, like, and trust" (KLT) factor of your practice. It is an effective way to build new relationships; strengthen existing relationships with colleagues, clients, media, and vendors; and let them know what is happening in your practice. These channels are new ways of talking to existing and new patients online. Think of social media as a network of communication channels. Focus your efforts on leading people toward making a purchase, for example, booking a consultation, scheduling a treatment, or purchasing a product from your practice.

Relationships need to go both ways, which speaks to the heart of the disconnect with many brands and practices. Keep the human component in customer relationships. It cannot be all one sided; don't show your hand on what you want to get from them. You have to give something to get something. Start by listening rather than talking and responding instead of promoting. Consumers want to get to know your practice before they schedule a consultation. Enlightened clinic managers know how to focus on growing long-term relationships.

Setting a Budget

WENDYISM

Social media is not free, nor is it cheap anymore. Think about what your time is worth.

It is a mistake to think of social media as free because it does not cost anything to start a Facebook page. That is a common fallacy because your time is your most valuable resource. A campaign with the right tone and relevance can create affordable, meaningful audience engagement, when compared with the cost of traditional advertising. There are not many other ways to reach thousands of potential patients all over the world without spending a fortune on print, TV, and public relations. Social media is a more cost-effective strategy to define your brand, build your reputation, and bring in new patients. It is driven by word of mouth, resulting in earned media rather than paid media.

However, it does require commitment and resources. At some point, you may have to outsource this marketing strategy and have a search engine optimization (SEO) company handle optimization for you.

Make a list of everything you need to do social media well. You can try it yourself, but it may not look good or function well unless you put in the time. Someone has to shoot and edit video. Factor in staff time, because even if you hire a social media agency, they will need guidance from someone in the clinic to manage them and make sure that what they are posting is accurate, on brand, and will not get you into trouble.

Social media is not something that should just be delegated to whoever has some free time. It should be executed strategically and consistently by someone who gets it. If you don't like it, it will show. Everything online is about transparency, and consumers are acutely aware of when you do not sound authentic. Marketing interns, grad students, and medical students can make excellent freelancers because they are typically avid social media users, need money, and can do the job from their phones.

Consider the frequency of creating content, promoting your clinic via ads and boosted posts, and then determine how much you are willing to spend and go from there. There are many aspects of social media that require programmers, writers, and designers. Determine exactly what you need and get a few recommendations from colleagues and compare proposals. Do not sign a contract without a lawyer looking it over to make sure you are protected. Regrettably, there are a lot of sleazy Internet marketing agencies out there who prey on unsuspecting doctors. Make sure that if they bid to do your social media marketing, that they are going to do it properly. Insist on original content and have a project manager assigned to your account. All too often, these agencies will create a single blog post or landing page for a specific procedure, and use it for all of their clients, even those who are competitors in the same market. That should be a BIG red flag.

SOCIAL SAFETY

Always make sure your clinic owns all of your URLs—for websites, blogs, even your Facebook page. Keep copious records of all of your logins. If you terminate your contract with a web designer or social media consultant, change all passwords immediately to stay secure. Similarly, if you let an employee go or someone leaves in a suspicious way, change all the passwords ASAP!

Measuring Results

It is important to track where your clicks are coming from to stay on top of your social media results on a monthly basis. Analytics are readily available for most platforms so you can continually measure the response you get.

Facebook Insights are easy to use and reports can be created, which you can download and compare. You can go back years to measure success year over year, track best times of day and engagement, and figure out what the best measurement is for the strategy you are following—those are the numbers to pay the most attention to.

When tracked and tweaked regularly, a social media campaign can deliver excellent marketing dividends. The key to success is consistent measurement of the impact of your social efforts. With limited time and resources at your disposal, you need to know what is working and what is not.

The best way to assess the return on investment (ROI) for your social media marketing efforts is to track the number of website conversions that originated from your social media networks. Use Google Analytics to track how many people visit your website by clicking on the site content links that you post on social networks, or shaing your links with other users.

---

3 FREE TOOLS TO TRACK YOUR SOCIAL MEDIA

1. Facebook Insights
2. Twitter Analytics
3. Google Analytics, Google Alerts

Monitor the Most Significant Metrics

WENDYISM

Engagement is the true holy grail of social media.

Many people buy into the theory that the most valuable metric is the total number of followers your social network attracts. Although that is the logical number to pay attention to, it is far from the only one that counts. Equally important is the sustainability of the followers. Your social network should retain followers as it attracts new ones.

With many billions of people around the world using social media, it is a numbers game, and size does matter. Local relevance of your network membership is more important for aesthetic clinics. Conversions will usually happen only from the targeted, local audience in your case. If you are using paid advertising on social media, track the cost per lead or cost per follower generated. The increase in new patients or treatments should be enough to justify the advertising spend.

Social media result monitoring and measuring is an ongoing task, and you should be tracking the results on a weekly or at least a monthly basis.

Analyze Your Conversions

Set up customized goals for different types of conversions that you wish to track. Conversions or responses can come in various forms, such as a lead, an inquiry, a downloaded form or coupon, a subscription to your e-newsletter, or anything else that requires a specific action. Go to Traffic Sources to look for social conversion data, and click on "Conversions." Detailed instructions are available to guide you through setting up your social tracking goals.

SOCIAL MEDIA TIP SHEET

- Learn the nuances of platforms your patients are on and best practices to use them.
- Develop a monthly calendar for each platform you are active on.
- Allocate a budget for ads, promotions, boosted posts to generate awareness, and conversion of new patients.
- Create shareable content that is unique to each platform and user experience.
- Assign roles within your clinic to execute a comprehensive social media strategy.
- Enlist external vendors as needed for help with strategy, content creation, posting, Facebook/Instagram ad management.

Posting Guidelines

Ideal posting times will depend on who you are trying to reach. If you are in the city and people who work in offices are coming in to see you during their lunch hour, that time frame may make sense. The only way to really know is to change times and see where you get more engagement, and then figure out a strategy to maximize it.

The chart of Best Posting Cadence below is intended as a guideline only to keep it manageable, although there is no definitive rule. If you are tracking engagement as you should be, you will be able to tell if you are posting too frequently and fans are not engaging. The number of times you post plus the timing of your posts can spell success or failure. Certain days and times may be better than others, based on your target audience.

BEST POSTING CADENCE

Platform	Baseline (Keeping the Lights On)	Optimum (Best Practice)
Blog	Biweekly	Weekly
Facebook	Three times per week	Daily
Facebook LIVE	Biweekly	Weekly
Instagram	Daily	Twice daily
Instagram Stories	Weekly	Two to three times per week
LinkedIn	Weekly	Twice weekly
Pinterest	Twice weekly	Three times per week
Snapchat	Weekly	Two to three times per week
Twitter	Daily	Three times a day
YouTube	Weekly	Two times per week
Google+	Weekly	Two times per week

Do not feel pressure to post multiple times a day or even every day unless you have something that adds value to share (e.g., a useful tip, information about a new treatment, a special offer, clinic news, etc.). If you flood your followers' feeds with useless content, you risk losing them forever. Engagement will suffer, and they will start unfollowing you and lose interest in your brand.

6 RULES FOR SOCIAL SUCCESS

1. **Outsource what you cannot do effectively.** Do you have someone on staff who can do it well, and does he or she have time to manage multiple platforms consistently? When it becomes overwhelming, either hire a marketing intern to help or outsource your social media to an experienced agency.
2. **Track each tactic to measure success and return on investment (ROI).** To know what working or if a change of focus is needed or an increase in investment or time, resources, or staff, you need to track results.
3. **Know your target markets.** Do not waste time and money on tactics that will not resonate with your target audience. You can have a main target and also subtargets to expand your reach. Start by knowing who you want to attract and what you want to do more of (e.g., lasers, fillers, body shaping, or skincare services).
4. **Invest in training.** Give your team the right training to manage your digital marketing. The more they know, the more likely they will be successful.
5. **Make it easy for patients to find you.** Include social links on all signage and marketing materials from brochures to appointment cards and e-blasts, and place links above the fold on your website landing page.
6. **Consistency and clarity are key.** You won't see results from doing something once. Create a social media marketing plan for 12 months, by creating content one month at a time, use consistent themes, images, and hashtags that speak to your clinic brand.

Having a robust social media program is a critical success factor for aesthetic clinics. You may start out by relying on others for guidance and help. As you become more proficient, start experimenting on your own and branching out. As you get comfortable with social media, you will be more inclined to collaborate with strategic partners and work together to maximize results.

The biggest challenge is how well clinics can implement strategies to get the most benefits out of the effort. A well-executed social media strategy will enable your clinic to cut through the clutter and stand out from the crowd. With the advancements made in social media tracking platforms, you can properly measure the key performance indicators (KPIs) that are most important for your clinic. If your progress is not measured, you cannot set benchmarks and improve your results. Set metrics to determine what your goals are. For instance, if your main goal is to create a following, measure followers, fans, and subscribers. If you wish to generate traffic to your clinic website, set a metric for unique visitors generated from your social platforms.

Be Strategic about the Most Valuable Platforms (MVPs)

To get the most ROI from social media marketing, choose your platforms wisely. You don't need to be the first to jump on all of them. New platforms and mobile apps seem to crop up all the time, but that does not mean that they are worth your interest unless the users are among your target patient audience. For example, if your clinic mainly attracts patients interested in anti-aging treatments, you may do best on Facebook and Instagram.

Facebook is still the biggest of all platforms and the place to begin if you can only manage one. Instagram would be my number two. It is a must for aesthetic clinics and offers a valuable way to give customers a taste of your clinic experience. Twitter is a good way for businesses to interact with customers. YouTube is all video, which makes it more difficult for clinics to use without creating original content of their own.

Tell Patients How to Find You

The main target audience for your social media includes patients who already know you. But don't leave it up to chance that they will know how to find you on their own. Whenever possible, choose the same name across platforms for consistency, for example, @WendyLewisCo or @JonesAesthetics. Post social buttons on all other marketing materials, including website landing page, e-mail marketing, blog posts, brochures, invitations, print advertisements, newsletters, and appointment cards. Include social network links on each platform to connect with other platforms on which you are active. Add tabs on your Facebook page to link to Twitter, YouTube, Pinterest, and Instagram. Last, post a sign in an elegant frame at the front desk, waiting room, and in treatment rooms, so patients and guests can connect with you.

It Is Not All about You—It Is about Them

Learn the difference between talking at your fans and talking to them. Even if you have scores of followers, if you do not engage with them properly, it is a wasted effort. Avoid overposting content that is purely self-promotional, for example, *"The first clinic in the Midlands to…," "The Best Cosmetic Doctor in London,"* and so on. This content is neither clever nor imaginative, neither entertaining nor eye catching. Think of your social media platforms as places to share information, interests, and passions. By the same token, if every post is just about a "3 for 2 Offer" or "20% Off Fillers," fans will lose interest and eventually opt out, and you will have devalued your brand in the process.

Think about how best to engage with fans. What do they like? What are they looking for? What will they want to share? If you don't know, ask them. Use a survey or ask patients to give you some insights on what rocks their world.

Social media is a minefield for healthcare practitioners, so do not risk crossing any lines that may be blurred. Running a medical clinic is not the same as managing a retail shop or restaurant. We cannot play by the same rules. It presents many challenges for aesthetic clinics, but the rewards are there for those who are serious about it.

Social media is here to stay, and the sooner you accept it as a vital component of promoting your clinic's services and products, the faster you will be able to grow a fan and follower base. Design a strategy to address your goals over time, with the right people onboard, and a reasonable budget to see results. Do not get discouraged because you don't have thousands of Facebook fans in a month. Like SEO and any other marketing tactic, it takes time to move the needle.

The Community Manager Role

Social media offers instant access to positive or negative feedback, which provides valuable insights on the customer perspective. It also encourages creating relationships with prospective patients and customers before, during, and after they have booked a consultation or had a treatment in your clinic. This kind of intimate dialogue between brands and customers is something traditional advertising does not achieve. As patients interested in aesthetic treatments are increasingly seeking advice on social media platforms, a new role has evolved—that of the community manager.

This person can be in-house, or can also be a marketing consultant or external vendor who understands your brand and feels comfortable interacting with patients or customers. The community manager should be able to respond to simple requests in real time; redirect customers to your website, an e-mail address, or a phone number; and follow up if needed. In many cases, this person will act as the first point of contact on social media platforms, respond as messages come in or posts appear online. They are also tasked with alerting the practitioner as medical questions arise, or a more specific response is required.

Social media serves to establish a more personal relationship between practitioners and existing patients, as well as potential new patients. In addition to nurturing a more personal relationship with fans, a community manager acts as the voice of the clinic or brand.

With the staggering number of people and businesses active on social media channels, it is also getting harder for aesthetic practices to stand out in the digital world. It takes ingenuity and a creative mind-set to build a community and keep them engaged.

The traditional, one-way ad campaign has evolved into a more personal and dynamic two-way dialogue—the operative word being "two." Social media has facilitated this form of brand promotion and allows companies to connect and engage with their customers in unprecedented ways.

Social media is all about instant gratification. Therefore, socially active customers expect brands and companies to respond often, literally in real time. In this way, social media is transforming what was formerly referred to as customer relationship management (CRM). Consumers expect a response, and they want it *now* and usually on the same platform they used to reach out, such as Facebook Messenger, Twitter, e-mail, or your website. After 24 hours, it may be lost forever, and your clinic gets a black mark for being unresponsive.

This does not mean that traditional methods of communication (phone, e-mail, postal mail) have no place anymore. Clients today just want to be heard. They want to have a voice and connect with someone who gets them. They do not appreciate form letters, or "Dear (insert customer name)" e-mails. They can see right through these tactics.

They are also wise to robots and don't love them. On some clinic websites, "chatbots," as they are called, are used to substitute for a human to answer simple questions, such as "What are your clinic hours?" or "Do you offer laser hair removal?" However, a robot cannot replace a living, breathing person with a pulse who is able to connect with customers on a deeper level and offer empathy. Messenger apps do offer canned replies, scripted marketing jargon, and prewritten responses for business pages. Consumers can always tell when the entity called "Joe" or "Sue" on the other end of the chat screen is a robot. Messaging is morphing into a hybrid of live and digital communications. It is important to humanize these interactions, particularly when a patient is already mad at you.

Scheduling posts can be challenging for any busy practitioner. Set aside time to plan what you want to post and to schedule those posts. Assign a point person to be in charge of social media management. This can be a detailed and time-consuming endeavor. The type of person who is wel-suited for this task may not be a "nuts and bolts" person who excels with analytics and budgets. It is a different side of the brain at work. Those who excel at social media tend to be verbal, have with good communication skills, follow pop culture and current events, and a people person. If that is not you, enlist a staff member or hire an external vendor to take over the day-to-day scheduling, posting, and monitoring. If you hire a newbie, request a monthly content calendar for approval before any posts go live. This allows the practitioner or manager to oversee the social content and troubleshoot.

WENDYISM

Anyone assigned the task of interfacing with patients online should be fully onboarded to understand the nuances and limitations of an aesthetic practice and basic rules of patient privacy.

Engagement Strategies

People are more likely to engage with content that contains visuals, which includes photos, graphics, and video; and links. It could be a line drawing, but it has to be more engaging than just plain text. If you must just do text, at least break it up with hashtags and emojis to be more consumer friendly, and there is something of interest in it rather than just words.

Always attempt to create content that people care about and want to share. The more interesting your content is, the more engaging it will be. Posting endless updates about new products, sales, and special offers, or other promotional news won't cut it anymore. Social media users resent being blatantly sold to.

The ultimate goal is to give followers something that they actually want, and that they cannot get everywhere else. Informative, entertaining, and well-presented content updates with the right balance of words, hashtags, visuals, and links, is what it takes to grab their attention. Think about the types of content that appeal to you. Humor is always a good choice.

Social media engagement relies on daily interactions among users. While it is fine to use tools to help you with the burdensome task of posting, engaging with your audiences in real time is still the most effective way to grow your audience. So, use automatic posting platforms to help you with the basics, but do not rely on this tactic for all of your social media channels. For example, Facebook allows you to schedule drafts and posts, which can be a major timesaver.

It is acceptable to repost content more than once, especially if it performed well, but even if it did not. You can also repurpose your content by changing a graphic or a link or tweaking the words and hashtags. It may reach fans and followers at different times, in different time zones, or on different days of the week. You may find that just making a few small changes will get better engagement.

Determine the voice that your presence on each platform should have. In most cases, it will be from the practice as a whole. In some cases, the physician may want to post his or her own content in the first person. If someone engages on your page, make sure to reply in a timely fashion. Reply with links to other posts or invite them to follow or connect with your network. Retweet or share interesting posts that may be relevant to your followers. Social media is about sharing and keeping your platforms updated and current, and each platform has a specific user who wants to get content in a specific way.

The most effective time devoted to social media should be spent responding to and engaging with others. If you are not engaging with people, you are missing out on the marketing value of social media. Using these platforms solely for streaming content in a robotic fashion, the real point of the social aspect of social media will be lost.

To determine if your content is on the right track, monitor, monitor, monitor. Consistent tracking will enable you to identify the most effective social channels and to analyze the kind of content that gets the best engagement and response in the form of comments, likes, and shares. Invest maximum efforts in those areas to enhance the social engagement to a greater level. Better engagement can eventually result in more conversions.

There is no one-size-fits-all solution for converting followers from social networks to real clients. It is a long-term process, and the goal must be to build sustainable relationships with your network. Rather than aiming at quick sales, long-term relationships will produce greater benefits in terms of actual conversions.

4 STEPS TO ENGAGEMENT

Step 1: Choose your platforms
Create profiles on all relevant platforms and create your own clinic blog. Do not become active on any platform unless you are ready to make a commitment to posting, monitoring, and engaging with followers.

Step 2: Connect with your audience
Start connecting with colleagues, partners, professional organizations, and vendors. Encourage them to share your content with their networks to grow your online presence, which, in turn, will help to increase your SEO ranking—how high your clinic website will appear organically in search results—the higher your ranking, the more visible you are.

Step 3: Develop strong content
Be constant in your posting—once every day or once or twice a week. The frequency will depend on resources and time available, and should be established in your social media marketing plan. Share engaging posts, clever graphics, and video of interest to your target audience. Link your social media accounts so posts will be shared on individual feeds. Use a dashboard tool such as Hootsuite, which allows you to manage all your online platforms in one place by scheduling posts and sharing content (see section entitled Social Tools, this chapter on page 70).

Step 4: Engage with your network
Keep your network engaged. If someone replies or posts on any of your pages, ensure that you respond in a timely manner—under 3 hours at maximum. Reply with links to articles containing relevant information or videos that correspond with the user's query, or helpful links to your clinic pages, or invite them connect with your network.

Position Yourself as an Authority

As an aesthetic practitioner, you want to be the go-to person who your fans can trust to get fair and balanced information on topics that matter to them. All the clutter online makes people want to focus on people or entities who give them what they want. Your followers should know to turn to you as a voice of expertise in aesthetic medicine. Consumers are wary about aggressive marketing messages, but they will trust experts.

People want to see a glimpse of who a practitioner is in real life, and sharing a little about who you are is a good thing. However, try to avoid oversharing too many personal details of your life. Once you put it out there, you can never reel it back in.

Shareable Content

The key to success is to consistently produce good content that is easy to share and to continue a dialogue. Use your content to identify fans who will talk about your practice and what you have done for them; discover what they love about you and what you can do to motivate them to share that love. You will never get your followers to talk about you by only talking at them. Social tools give you the means to ask them questions, invite them to take part in the content creation process, and give them a sense that they have a stake in your brand. This is the core of what you are trying to achieve.

I see a lot of really good content from clinics on social media, but I also see a lot of content that misses the mark. One reason is that practitioners are severely restricted on how creative they can get. After all, you are not selling lipsticks, shoes, or gourmet pizza. You have to keep your medical hat on and think very differently than other service businesses to reach your target audiences. Aesthetic clinics are looking for a very specific, niche market, and targeting is an important part of marketing when you consider the money and resources required to do it right.

Targeting is essential. The more narrowly you target, the more effective you will be, and the less money it will cost you in the end. Assess the platforms that are the most relevant to your patient population. In most cases it is going to be Facebook, Instagram, Twitter, and YouTube. It could be Snapchat if you have a younger population, depending on where you are located. Figure that out first, start with Facebook, Instagram, Twitter (F.I.T.) (see Chapter 8), and expand as you need to.

Content curation is easier and faster. Post interesting content on your social networks, and pull the trigger. Getting followers to share your content with their followers means making sure your content aligns with your brand and interests your audience.

Another benefit is increasing web traffic. The more social media shares you receive, the higher your search ranking will be.

Tailor Content to the Platform

Each platform has a specific type of user. Everyone has their own favorites that they spend more time on, and they consume content in very different ways. The format varies substantially, so you have to figure out how your content is going to look on Twitter, if you have it automated, or on every other platform if you plan to share it.

I am not a big fan of duplicating content on multiple channels, but content can be reformatted. You can use the same basic content by repackaging it in a way that will fit other platforms and appeal to that set of users.

WHAT GOES WHERE

Network	Content Specs
Facebook	*It might look scary, but the results are amazing! At the Smith Clinic, we use state-of-the-art nonablative lasers for melasma and pigmentation. Dr. Smith recommends 2–3 treatments spaced about 1 month apart for a smoother and more even-toned complexion. #beautifulskinstartshere*
	Since Facebook allows you to write more copy, you can elaborate in posts and add before/after photos or a video of Jane's treatment.
Instagram	*How gorgeous is Jane's skin after her laser treatment?! #beautifulskin*
	Note the difference in tone, the exclamation point; more colloquial, conversational; targeting a younger audience of users who are all about compelling visuals.
YouTube	*Dr. Smith will perform a laser treatment on Jane to reduce her sun damage, pigmentation, lines, and wrinkles...*
	Factual and focused how-to video; demonstrate expert care and professionalism to educate viewers on how the treatment works and what they can expect to drive awareness.
LinkedIn	*According to XYZ organization, laser resurfacing was the third most popular treatment performed in 2017 based on consumer demands...*
	Very professional tone used—you are talking to colleagues, vendors, and business partners—you are not talking directly to consumers.
Pinterest	*Flawless younger-looking skin after a laser resurfacing treatment.*
	More relatable, causal, unique, and searchable content that is inspirational and results oriented, with before/after photo.
Snapchat	*Jane hates her sun damage from years at the beach, so Dr. Smith is going to give her a laser treatment...*
	Experiential video content inviting the viewer to get a sneak peek behind the curtain of your aesthetic clinic.
Twitter	*Got brown spots? Learn how laser treatments reversed Jane's pigmentation bit.ly/lasersforpigment #beautifulskinstartshere*
	Use Twitter as a conduit to direct the user to another platform of your choice where you can elaborate on laser treatments with additional text, and add video or an image to the post.
Google+	*Join our circle to learn about what lasers can do for your skin.*
	Google+ is still in flux, but it is an important platform and not one you can afford to overlook because Google owns it. Most practices use it mainly for SEO, not as a social network.

10 WAYS TO ENHANCE YOUR POSTS

1. Original snapshots
2. Before/after photos
3. Links to website, articles, blogs, podcasts
4. Short videos
5. Original graphics with clinic branding
6. Infographics
7. Quotagraphics
8. Memes, GIFs
9. Slide presentations
10. Infographics

COPYRIGHT INFRINGEMENT WARNING

DO NOT just lift any images, visuals, or patient photos from Google, a public website, or another clinic's site. This practice may result in copyright infringement that can end up in legal action being taken against the doctor, the clinic, or the individual.

You may also license appropriate images as needed. Stock photography sites offer a vast library of images, vectors, illustrations, and videos of varying quality that can be tweaked to make them your own. Try to avoid using the same popular stock images of women's faces that can be seen all over the Internet. Select images that are fresh and modern, without dated hair and makeup, and look more realistic and relatable for your customers. The most economical way to use these sites is through a monthly or annual subscription where images can be licensed literally for pennies in some cases. There is also a plethora of royalty-free images available. Use the Advanced Image Search function on Google Images to look for images that are "free to use or share, even commercially."

STOCK IMAGE SITES

Stock Images Subscriptions	Royalty-Free Images
Bigstockphoto.com	Picabay.com
Corbisimages.com	Unsplash.com
Creativemarket.com	Deathtostock.com
Depositphotos.com	Gratisography.com
Fotolia.com	
Fotosearch.com	
Istockphoto.com	
Shutterstock.com	

WENDYISM

Stimulating User-Generated Content (UGC)—Real patients talking about you and their first-hand experience in your clinic—is the ultimate goal.

Poster's Block

So, what do you do when you are just not feeling it?

The pressure of a blank status update staring you in the face is a common lament. For community managers, this can be a real dilemma because they always want to be creative, interesting, and on brand. Sometimes you just have nothing cool to say.

Avoid getting stuck in a rut by creating a slew of content (1 week to 1 month's worth) at a time. Leave room for extra posting as topics and news arise. Check out my list of platforms and apps that make it easier to schedule in advance and automate some of your posting (see page 92). Make sure to intersperse scheduled content with fresh, timely comments, replies, questions, and so on.

8 STRATEGIES TO GET YOUR JUICES FLOWING

1. **Smart data mining:** Comments and discussions on Facebook and LinkedIn are social media gold. They offer insights into what your audience cares about. Use these clues to spark new conversations. Ask questions; people love to talk about themselves.
2. **Unleash your inner news junkie:** The news is great fodder for picking up on a theme that is trending to tie into your content. Set Google or Yahoo! alerts for topics that may be suitable for commenting on or sharing. Stay on top of celebrity happenings your audience follows.
3. **Let's get personal:** Do not be afraid to reveal a few details about the people in your clinic. Users love anecdotes that draw them in so they feel part of your brand. Give them a glimpse of your clinic by opening the curtain a little.
4. **Amplify media coverage:** Media hits offer great material for social media platforms and blogs. They can be repackaged in different ways for each channel. An appearance on local news can be used as a link on your Facebook page, a clip for YouTube (if you have the rights to post it), or a recap for a blog post. Media hits also tend to get shared.
5. **Be a good listener:** Brands often tell the story they want their audiences to hear, without considering what they are really interested in. To stay relevant, watch what your audience is talking about and the questions that pop up. Use this as a framework for key messages to weave into your content.
6. **Let me entertain you:** A dose of humor never hurt anyone. Creating engaging content infuses an upbeat, lighthearted tone that can awaken your audience. Anecdotes and real-life stories (*not* about patients!) can make your content more interesting. Cool visuals are also of huge importance.
7. **Make it actionable:** Is the content you are posting enabling your audience to learn or get something that they cannot get somewhere else? Are you talking about something they want to know more about? Is your content offering personal insights to help them make good choices? Create content that leads your audience to a course of action they can follow.
8. **What's the point?:** The content you create should have a point. It can be geared toward gaining insights into what your community thinks. Use a subtle way to extract nuggets of information to find out what they need to know to try your services. The more you know about your audience, the better you can keep them interested and engaged.

Make every post count. Before you post, take the time to get the content right so it comes across as real and sincere to have the most effect.

BASIC FORMAT TYPES

Platform	Content Format
Blog	Paragraph of 500 words approximately, image or video
Facebook	Paragraph, link, video or image, emojis, hashtags
Google+	Snippet, image or video, hashtags
Instagram	Image or video, snippet, emojis, hashtags
LinkedIn	Paragraph, image, link, tags
Pinterest	Image, pin boards, optimized with search terms, hashtags
Snapchat	Video, emojis, hashtags
YouTube	Original video, snippet, optimized with search terms, hashtags
Twitter	280 characters, add a link, image or video, hashtag

How to Create Clever Hashtags

Hashtags are a must-have component of social media marketing. A hashtag is a symbol (#) with a phrase that is searchable. Hashtags are used throughout all or most social platforms and are mandatory on Facebook, Instagram, and Twitter.

Don't go crazy creating random or branded hashtags. Unless you have a budget to promote these, for a contest or public relations campaign, they will be ownable but not searchable. You may use a hashtag for your clinic and/or practice, such as #AskDrB. (We often use #WLCO for our company posts.)

You are better off using the most popular relevant hashtags, because these will get more eyes on your content. Choose some key hashtags to use frequently, then add more for specific content, and pay attention to what is trending. If you choose hashtags that are too general or obscure, your content may not show up because it is not searchable.

Staying on top of trending hashtags is also useful to join the conversation and to create a bridge between your clinic brand and customers. Instagram users are the biggest fans of hashtags, and you will often see posts that are literally all hashtagged terms, thus rendering them unreadable. If that is your strategy, your photos must be totally gorgeous to attract the readers' attention. Blurry photos taken on your phone, or pictures out of context with poor angles and lighting are as bad as, if not worse than, no visuals at all. Social media users have high standards for photos—most especially on Instagram.

Only use hashtags on posts that are relevant to the topic or they lose their value. For example, if you use general but super popular hashtags, like #Instagood (613 million), #instadaily (280 million), and #beautiful (400 million), your post will not generate engagement because these are too vague to matter for your brand.

Emoji Nation

Today there are emojis that represent every person, place, or thing on the planet, and nearly everyone is using them to create more entertaining conversations and personal interactions on mobile platforms. Apparently, people like face emojis best.

Do not just choose your emojis (or words for that matter) randomly. They should be relatable and relevant to both the content and the user. They have to make sense to communicate with users on their level. If you want to connect with millennials, it means mastering the art of speaking emoji.

Emojis are used to convey a lot of information with as few words as possible. But don't forego words entirely. You need a balance of both to get your message across. Try incorporating a few relevant emojis (three to five) that accurately express the intended meaning to see how your audience responds before going emoji-crazy.

Since emojis are a staple of our day-to-day conversation across text messages and social media platforms, they can help make your practice feel more human. Brands that showcase their personalities may be better able to create lasting and trusted connections with followers by resonating with them on a more personal level. Emoji usage adds to eye-catching messages by inciting an emotion that may lead to a consultation, treatment, or connection.

Emojis have their origins in Japanese culture, and apparently a whole lot of meaning can get lost in translation. To stay safe and risk offending anyone, avoid anything that could be misconstrued as being sexual or offensive, such as a hot dog, peach, cherries, beads of sweat, or a mound of feces, to name a few. Think of these symbols as a way to add to the content rather than just replacing words. Use emojis at the end of a written sentence to add some color. For the most part, they act like exclamation points, providing cues about how to understand the words that came before them. If you are using a string of emojis to tell a story, they should also be placed in the proper order or timeline.

If you are not entirely sure what the hidden meaning of an emoji is, look it up. But even if you know the true meaning, the intended recipients may have no idea. Stick with the commonly used emojis, and occasionally experiment with something more unique to see how your followers respond.

Whereas emojis are powerful, if your text is filled with characters, but when the user clicks on it the user is directed to a nonresponsive, mobile-unfriendly, or outdated page, adding the right smileys is not going to save you. Everything needs to integrate seamlessly.

EMOJIS DEFINED

- Emojipedia.com
- Emojisaurus.com

Social Tools

The best way to effectively manage multiple social media platforms is to employ social media management tools that can improve your efficiency and turbocharge your analytics and results. Although this is not always considered best practice, for busy aesthetic clinics, these essential tools offer myriad benefits for organization, scheduling, sharing, and analytics.

SOCIAL MEDIA MANAGEMENT TOOLS

- Hootsuite
- Sprout Social
- Buffer
- TweetDeck
- Social Oomph
- IFTTT
- BuzzSumo
- CoSchedule
- Sendible
- Socialbakers

Your best bet for choosing a social media management tool is based on how deeply involved you want to become with social media. If you need the best time-saving features, I have found Hootsuite to be comprehensive with excellent customer service. Most of these have free introductory services and then upgrades for access to additional features from there. If you are serious about social media, you should spring for the basic paid version to get started. As you add platforms, you may want to upgrade.

To date, none of these services offer the ability to schedule and post directly to Instagram, but hopefully that will change in the near future as everyone is clamoring for it.

8

F.I.T.: Facebook, Instagram, Twitter

A large social-media presence is important because it's one of the last ways to conduct cost-effective marketing. Everything else involves buying eyeballs and ears. Social media enables a small business to earn eyeballs and ears.

Guy Kawasaki

WENDYISM
Think of Facebook, Instagram, Twitter (F.I.T.) as the triple header of social media platforms.

These three platforms integrate seamlessly and are a must for aesthetic practitioners finding their way into social media marketing.

Facebook is the number one global social media network. It is a virtual meeting ground where friends, family, and colleagues come to read what you choose to share. With more than two billion monthly users worldwide, Facebook has become an essential component of a clinic marketing program. Aesthetic clinics can build brand loyalty, establish the expertise of their medical staff, engage with patients on a deeper level, and drive traffic to their clinic website.

For clinics new to social media, Facebook is the place to begin. Your customized Facebook business page can feature your product and service offering, highlight multiple locations, provide appointment scheduling, offer monthly specials, and grow a fan base. Your page can be promoted via e-mail blasts, Facebook ads, promoted posts, and your Facebook network of fans directly. Content sharing also means having Share buttons on your website and blog for social media optimization purposes to encourage visitors to share your content.

Facebook is a great tool to raise your practice's profile and connect with like-minded people. It should be integrated into your overall marketing efforts. The best Facebook approaches complement rather than replicate your practice website or blog—meaning that both sites should have fresh content on them, relative to each audience. Use Facebook as a platform to share engaging content on a variety of topics that could be of interest to your "fans." You will need to make a commitment to being active on Facebook in terms of posting and engaging with your "fans" or "friends." Like search engine optimization (SEO), social media takes time to see results—sometimes 3–6 months.

The potential audience for your practice on Facebook is huge. Current patients and clients may "like" your page, and by this recommendation, their friends will also be made aware of your business. Fans can write comments on your page, such as queries about your products or services, news items that are being shared, or their success stories for other customers to see. Your Facebook business page is a powerful way to interact with your fans and potential customers. Keep listening and engaging with your audience to understand what people are thinking about your product or service. Facebook is a great way to improve relationships and listen to your audience for clues on how to elevate your service.

To generate excitement, content should incorporate anyone who can endorse you or provide testimonials and enter the conversation. Posts should be fresh, creative, and interesting to capture the users' attention.

Setting Up Your Business Page

Business pages are where the information about your clinic posted. Posts should include all of the key messages on your clinic website landing page, products and treatments offered, special training, awards, and information about the practitioners.

WHAT YOU NEED TO KNOW

- Design a cover photo of 850 × 315 pixels.
- Create a video for your cover photo.
- Select a square profile picture of at least 180 pixels in width.
- Choose a pinned post to showcase top content.
- Decide which apps to feature prominently on your timeline.
- Set milestones for current or past dates. Milestone images are 843 × 403 pixels.

Brand page cover pictures are not clickable; text links here may confuse fans. These images can be changed, rotated, or updated as often as you want to keep the page fresh. Facebook also allows customized videos instead of still images for page cover photos.

As always, Facebook has strict guidelines for what cover images may not contain:

- Price or purchase information, such as "40% off" or "Download it at our website"
- Contact information, such as web address, e-mail, mailing address, or other information intended for your page's About section
- References to user interface elements, such as Like or Share, or any other Facebook site features

Facebook also stipulates that you cannot "encourage or incentivize people."

The profile picture sits with the top half laid over the cover picture, so use contrast to showcase the profile image. Use a square image for best results.

Make sure the categories you selected are the most applicable. (From your page, click "Edit Info" to be able to review and edit your Basic Information page.) If you choose the general category called "Companies & Organizations," a possible second-tier category of "Health/Medical/Pharmaceuticals" might be a suitable choice. If you choose general category "Local Businesses & Places," then the second-tier "Hospital/Clinic" may be a better choice. Select the most relevant options so patients and colleagues can find you in as few clicks as possible.

Creating a unique URL helps you to get found more easily and direct people to your page. For example, our URL for our global beauty site Beautyinthebag.com's page is facebook.com/Beautyinthebag. Once you choose a unique URL, you will need permission to change it.

The Administration panel will help you manage your page. Use it to view statistics, social insights, and a log of your own activity as you grow your page. You are also able to assign page roles such as Admins and Editors. This is the preferred way to give staff and vendors access to your page, rather than allowing them to log into Facebook using your account details. If the relationship goes south, as an Admin, you can remove them as Editors on the page, thereby rescinding any access.

Adding Apps

Take full advantage of adding custom applications to the top of your page. Apps let you highlight specific areas of focus beyond the basic information on your main page, like subpages so that fans can learn more about each service line, and view embedded videos. You could also use apps to post additional locations and job openings, or share information about upcoming events or announcements. Choose other apps to highlight to allow for a greater level of personalization. Within these apps, users can learn more about all of the services, products, and treatments you offer and view embedded videos. You may also create secondary pages, such as for additional clinics, allied practitioners, and locations. The goal is to display your best content or elements that keep users engaged and that get them to stay on the page.

Your clinic Facebook page should include all the information a new client would need to make a decision to try or buy.

FACEBOOK'S CALL TO ACTION

Facebook integrated a call to action (CTA) on pages that are free to use, at least for now. CTAs help drive people from Facebook to take action such as booking appointments or making a purchase.

To add a CTA button to your page, Go to your Page's Cover Photo and click on Create Call-to-Action.

There are five CTA buttons to choose from:

1. **Shop Now**—Promote a new product or treatment, special offer, or limited edition
2. **Learn More**—Showcase a new blog post, direct visitors to your website or microsite
3. **Sign Up**—Enroll for a newsletter, blog, event, webinar, or mailing list
4. **Book Now**—Book an appointment or schedule a treatment
5. **Download**—Promote e-books and white papers, brochures, and special offers

Choose your CTA and the Destination URL that you want to link to (e.g., your website home page, blog, or specific landing page). Facebook also allows you to track your clicks to the CTA you have chosen to see how it is working, and this can be changed at any time.

Likable Posts

Pictures of faces, especially eyes and lips, capture attention because they are nice to look at, and there is eye contact. Content should be light—and have a positive tone. If you are trying to market a medical spa or a clinic, lose some overly technical or clinical language. Keep it professional in that you are talking to prospective patients and media, but avoid any kind of complicated words and descriptors that require lengthy explanations, words that are hard to spell, or phrases that will not be picked up by a search engine.

Choose your content themes judiciously. Politics is off limits, especially in the current world climate. With sex, you have to be careful as a healthcare practitioner. Avoid posting and reacting to anything that could be misconceived or that someone could potentially take offense to. However, on Facebook you are able to go back and edit the post if needed. In general, ascribe to the adage, "When in doubt, leave it out."

Facebook gives you a lot more room to work with as opposed to Twitter where you have 280 characters, and Instagram on which a short intro copy is more typically used. However, if you don't capture your reader in the first sentence or two, he or she is not going to read any more, so posts that are too long are not ideal because fans may not click on them. Three or four lines is a good length, and the most important things should appear front and center.

Plain text does not perform well on Facebook. Try to make it look as magazine-like as possible. Visually interesting and appealing posts work best. Experiment with different types and formats of content to see what generates the best results. Avoid repetitive content on Facebook. If you are going to post on Monday, do not post something similar on Tuesday. Mix it up to keep it interesting.

Avoid posting only information about your clinic, practitioners, promotions, or specials. Include other content that will be relevant to your fans across a wider range of topics.

12 BEST CONTENT BUCKETS

- Anti-aging
- Beauty trends
- Bridal
- Celebrity news
- Fashion
- Fitness and nutrition
- Hair-loss
- Health and wellness
- Patient safety
- Statistics
- Seasonal themes
- Skincare tips

Growing Your Fan Base

To build up a base of fans and followers to market to, engage with others in your own field and related fields, and your community, in order to cross-promote your social media efforts and expand your audience. Aim for alliances with people who have bigger followings than you do, but have a similar target audience of consumers with common interests, such as beauty, health, wellness, fitness, and skincare.

Follow colleagues, affiliates, partners, and neighboring businesses on social media. It is a great way to show support for their businesses, too. You should also follow brands and vendors you work with, suppliers, manufacturers, and distributors, as well as organizations you belong to, universities, and institutions you are connected with.

On the right side of your Facebook page, under Community, there is a tab called Invite Your Friends to Like This Page. Use this feature to invite people you already know and are connected with (*not* patients) to like your business page and build a fan base.

Geo-Targeting

Geo-targeting is an effective way to segment your message to target a specific audience or demographic based on their location—country, state, or city. Facebook and Twitter feature tools that allow you to share the right kind of content to your audience. Instagram also has this feature on their Sponsored Post ad platform.

With Facebook Insights, you can also learn the locations, dominant languages, ages, and gender among your social media audience. This knowledge can help you cater campaigns to specific target audiences, which will provide a better return on investment (ROI). The more targeted your campaigns, the more effective and less expensive they will be, with a lower margin for error.

Another way to use geo-targeting is to like and friend local businesses and community organizations in your market who are more likely to friend and follow you back because they are familiar with your practice.

Facebook Ad Strategies

If you noticed a decline in how many Facebook fans have been viewing and interacting with your organic posts over the past few years, you are not alone. Until about 5 years ago, every time you posted content on your Facebook page, approximately 16% of your fans would see your update. Fast forward to now, and only about 2% of your fans will ever lay eyes on your content. The new algorithms have slashed organic reach down to single digits, which makes it more expensive to grow your fan base.

One reason for this is that there is so much content being put out on Facebook that news feeds are overloaded, which makes getting eyes on your posts far more competitive. Facebook is also trying to show users the content that is most relevant to them, so some content gets screened out automatically. Similarly, organic posts on Instagram have dropped to the bottom of users' feeds, which has made it next to impossible to grow followers without some investment in sponsored posts.

Facebook is the premier social platform to keep up with loyal patients and attract new ones through targeted ads and boosted posts. Of all the social channels in play, Facebook offers a highly sophisticated advertising platform that is widely considered the gold standard. It allows you to create targeted ads for different audiences, set a daily or campaign budget, and measure the results across devices.

Best practices are to test different types of targeting to find the most responsive audience to which to promote your clinic services. Experiment with interest categories, friends of followers, and website audience lookalikes. Try these tactics in separate ad sets to determine which will deliver the best results for your brand.

FACEBOOK AD TARGETING TIPS

- **Do not target too broadly**—Narrow your audience by adding only one key interest category at a time. For example, start with "Ghent Cosmetic Lasers" and then broaden this category after you have run your campaigns for a week or two, adding "BOTOX Ghent" or "BOTOX, Facial fillers Ghent," and so on.
- **Target by city, zip or postal code, or region**—If your clinic is mostly local, target your audience by their zip or postal code. This can also be helpful if you know that a specific city or zip code offers good conversion rates. Identify the cities/areas that convert well in Google Analytics in the "Audience Insights" section.
- **Test images first, then copy**—Images are a critical success factor for ad performance, second only to copy. If you are not getting results, switch out the image first to test it. If that does not help, change the copy as well. Keep trying different combinations until you get the traction you want.
- **Use action words**—Tell your fans what you want them to do. For example, "download an e-book," "schedule a consultation," "sign up for our newsletter," or "RSVP to a seminar."
- **Use your connections**—Target people who are either connected or not connected to your Facebook page. If you want to reach a new audience, select "not connected to your Facebook Page." If you have an offer or new product, select "connected to your Facebook Page" to reach people who already know your brand.
- **Create custom audiences**—Facebook lets you upload customer e-mail addresses or other identifiers to build your own audience targeting. This strategy can be very effective and may be best managed by a digital agency for best results.
- **Try lookalike audiences**—This allows you to target people based on data from fans of your Facebook page. Take your top 10 best customers, search their e-mail addresses and names on Facebook. Go to their Likes and create a spreadsheet of common interests. Look for any similar Likes across your top customers to know whom to target.

Boosting a Post

Because of the way Facebook works, most of the content you post is not going to be seen by very many people. Boosting posts so more of your target audience see it in their newsfeeds—for example, women in the United Kingdom aged 25–45 who like beauty, cosmetics, Botox, or lasers—is an affordable viable tactic that moves the needle. This may cost $20, or you can spend thousands if you want. But Facebook will show you exactly how many people you could be reaching at that level. If you spend $75, you may be able to reach 3,000–20,000 people who fall within that target audience.

The more targeted you can be, the better. You can target by geographical area, gender, level of education, marital status, shopping and lifestyle preferences, and more. It is a small investment, but in my experience, it really works. Without boosting your content, you may get discouraged by a lack of engagement because your posts will not be seen by the majority of your fans.

Contests and Competitions

Contests and competitions can help grow your fan base, but this strategy will not move the needle for your bottom line unless the participants are targeted so they are among the audience that you want to reach who can convert to become paying patients.

Generally, it is best to postpone these tactics until you have a sufficient following to market to. For some clinics, that may mean 500, for others it may be 1,000 or more. Dreaming up clever competitions and essay or photo contests to generate excitement online is a good way to test the waters. Everyone loves to have the chance to win something. But you may end up with 25 or 50 entries, some of whom may be serial contest entrants. If you do go there, set aside an ad budget to promote your contest through Facebook ads and boosted posts.

Instagram Strategy

Instagram is a free app (like Snapchat) to be downloaded from Apple Store or Google Play to use it. The network, which Facebook owns, is almost entirely mobile. There is a web version, but you cannot take photos or create new posts, and other functions are limited.

The app allows users to post their own photos and videos regram content of interest to their followers. As on Twitter, hashtags function as subjects for each post and provide a link to related posts that use the same hashtag. But Instagram is based mainly on photo and video posts and requires someone or something to take photos of, other than before and after photos of patients. This can include photos of your clinic, community events, your clinic or brand represented at exhibitions, your team, award ceremonies, a staff birthday, and/or any other snapshots that lend themselves to creating attractive images. Instagram users are elitists when it comes to photos; only the best and most attractive images will get liked and shared, so keep that in mind when selecting what to post.

Instagram is getting bigger, more important, and influential. To succeed with Instagram, choose someone to manage your content who has a good eye for detail and at least basic photography skills so that the images are high quality. You need to be creative. If you have amateurish, blurry, unappealing pictures on Instagram, they will not get regrammed, and people will unfollow you. To ace Instagram, you need to have some style and good taste and a clever mind, and know how to manipulate images.

On Instagram, you can tell your brand's story in a creative and visually appealing way. Therefore, it is important to consider how Instagram fits into your overall brand marketing strategy before taking the plunge. Is your objective to increase awareness, shift perception, or reach a new audience? Who will manage Instagram? What subjects will make interesting posts? How will you represent your brand?

The Instagram Mystique

Instagram is a place to discover, have fun, and be inspired. Users see curations of individual moments, experiences, and elements throughout the world. The Instagram community expects brands to showcase their own moments, experiences, and elements that are transformative and aspirational. They are passionate about authenticity and insist on transparency.

Facebook has more text that requires more reading, whereas Twitter, Instagram, and Snapchat are short-content platforms. Experimenting and to be the first to know and the first to use are qualities that rank high among Instagram users. Instagram users can be celebrity obsessed, and feel connected to celebrities because they can directly communicate with them on their phones.

Visuals add a dimension to content that words alone cannot always convey. Instagram provides a platform to change, personalize, and share photos taken with your phone. It allows you to enhance colors, add filters or a frame, and share photos with other Instagram users and on social media platforms like Twitter and Facebook. It is the most important real-time photo-sharing platform, despite many others. Instagram is effective as a platform for talking about beauty products, cosmetics, skincare, as well as places, events, and travel. You can essentially tell your brand's story in a creative and visually appealing way, using photos, graphics, or videos.

Consider how this platform will fit into your overall brand marketing strategy. What is your objective? Are you interested in reaching a new, younger patient segment? Are you looking to raise your profile and increase awareness? The next question is what kind of content you plan to post, where you will get it, who can create the visuals needed, and who will manage Instagram postings. Getting the whole staff involved is the best way to make Instagram work for an aesthetic practice.

Instagrammers are posting, liking, and sharing primarily on their smartphones. Another distinction is that you will be posting on Instagram in real time primarily, although you have the ability to upload drafts to be posted at a later date and time. This is important if you are posting about an event or presentation—you need to post while it is still going on or it loses its impact and relevance.

Your Instagram strategy comes down to what your goals are and who your target customers are. If you are not utilizing Instagram in your clinic marketing, you are missing out on huge potential traffic and business.

Your Clinic on Instagram

Your Instagram profile is where people will look to find out more about your clinic. Instagram only gives you a maximum of 150 characters to explain your practice, so be concise, clear, and strategic in choosing your words. Add your location, a brief description, and a link to your website. If the account is in the name of the practice rather than the doctor, it may be best to use your logo or a graphic symbol. If it is in the doctor's name, you can use a headshot. Keep in mind that it will be cropped into a thumbnail-sized image and viewed on a smartphone screen. Add Twitter/Facebook/Snapchat names, and connect your Instagram to your Facebook page.

Getting started on Instagram is pretty much like other platforms, but it has a language and culture all its own. The challenge for healthcare practitioners is that it is all about visuals and videos. Text is used much more selectively, and often in the form of a string of catchy Instagram-specific hashtags. Using relevant, searchable, popular hashtags helps get your content found and followed. Stay vigilant to avoid posting any patient photos without express written consent, whether in the clinic, before and after procedures, or at a patient seminar.

To get active on Instagram, you have to follow other users, like their photos, and share their content. To start using Instagram, engage by following others who know you, liking their photos, and commenting on their posts. Next, announce to your fans and followers that you are on Instagram and go.

Optimize Your Profile

Your Instagram profile is like your business card, and it is where users will look to find out more about you and your clinic.

Set up your account and add the URL of your clinic website that will hyperlink to your landing page. Try to get the name as close to your business name as possible so that your brand is easily recognizable across all social media platforms.

The must-haves for your profile are as follows:

- High-resolution photo or image 150 × 150 pixels
- Brief description of your clinic
- A link back to your clinic website URL

You can use your logo, but it will be cropped into a circle and appear pretty small on most phones.

Engaging with Instagrammers

To engage with other Instagrammers, tag any brands, like skincare products or lasers, included in your photo. This will increase the likelihood that they will share the photo with their followers. Include the location of your photo or video when it helps tell the story of the image. To respect patients' right to privacy, *do not* tag patients or post photos or videos of patients without their express written consent.

Another way to engage with other users is to like and comment on their photos, and of course to respond to comments on your own images. To create strategic relationships on Instagram, find the brands and people you enjoy and can learn from in your followers and follow them back.

Designing Content

Instagram requires a fair amount of upkeep. You need to include a caption, emojis, and at least five hashtags, but many users go for 20 per post. If you sell products in your practice, they are perfect to use in images to put on Instagram. A product in a beautiful setting, or a lovely smooth forehead would be fine.

The way to attract your target market is with content that connotes a compelling and inspiring story that makes people want to get on board with your brand and learn more. Don't be afraid to mix it up a little, and include images, videos, graphics, and memes. If you post the same kind of content every day, your feed will become boring, and followers will quickly lose interest.

Focus on what makes a provocative and eye-catching image (color, symmetry, form, balance, etc.). For example, don't just upload any old snapshot of skincare products; make it something "Insta-worthy" by adding a personal touch—show someone using the product, someone testing it on his or her hand, a collage of products with flowers and a shiny mirror, the product with a textural background, or the product in a garden or held up against a backdrop of a city street scene. Instagram is all about the visuals, so aim to build a cohesive and reproducible brand identity. Use the same filters, add your logo or a border, and establish a style that is unique to your clinic brand. Entrust your Instagram to someone who has good taste, has an artistic eye, and gets who your target clients are and how to engage them.

Consumers really use the platform by scanning an image, so if they don't like the image, they won't engage with the post. This underscores how important nailing the visual is on this platform.

Most importantly, posts should always be engaging and creative, which are qualities inherent to the platform. Instagram was not designed for users to share images with a lot of text obscuring them. It was created so people could share beautiful, original imagery.

Monitor how your content is doing as you go along. Key performance indicators (KPIs) include likes, comments or engagement, and number of followers. Produce images and videos that are well crafted and feel like they were made for Instagram. Instagrammers have very high standards when it comes to visuals. Post photos and videos of beautiful and interesting happenings that also feel authentic and immediate; think in the moment. Videos can only be a maximum of 15 seconds, so these are just capturing a snippet of time. The more good content you post, the faster you can attract followers—the operative word being "good."

Posting daily is often considered best practice. Less than that and you lose momentum; more than that and you risk annoying followers by clogging up their feeds with things they are not interested in or do not want to see. For example, a picture of your new puppy or a staff member bringing her baby to the office may get a deluge of likes and comments, whereas a special deal on a filler may go practically unnoticed. It is all about how you package it. Pay attention to the engagement you get to gain a sense of what your followers really care about. Other popular themes are travel, great views, fashion, décor, food, art, and all things beauty.

WENDYISM

Be mindful that your goal is to engage—not enrage—your followers.

The keys to Instagram are creativity and inspiration, which is why, in my humble opinion, many practices have lost the plot. It is one thing to promote the occasional pictures of a lip filler, glycolic peel, tattoo removal, or even a cute rhinoplasty, but that is not really what Instagram is all about. If you are posting a stream of full body photos with pasties to cover nipples and private parts, this may be offensive to some people, or it may attract the wrong kind of followers.

Similarly, too much text on an image, a fuzzy or out of focus image, or a pixelated photo is sure to be overlooked. Instagrammers have an even shorter attention span than other social media users, and 100% of them are looking at their feeds on a mobile device because it is an app.

You can add up to 10 photos and videos to a single Instagram post, so users can swipe through to see each individual piece of content. These albums are a good way to combine photos and videos to tell stories and convey information in a more engaging way.

A useful feature within the Instagram platform is when you are about to post your message you have the option to have it automatically post immediately to Facebook and Twitter as well. This is a time saver, although it is not considered best practice.

Showcase Your Services and Products

Instagram is a cool way to show what you have to offer, but it cannot be all about you. Grow your followers by offering educational content, creative product shots or other posts of interest that are shareable.

---

10 INSTA IDEAS

1. Behind-the-scenes photos that followers cannot get on other platforms
2. Staff or team photos
3. Event photos or videos
4. Photos shared by your followers (with written permission)
5. Demos of services: spa treatment, consultation, injectables, etc.
6. Memes and GIFs
7. Boomerang of Slo-Mo videos
8. Clinic tours to showcase what you offer
9. Action shots of the doctor at work
10. Instagram Stories

Balance fun images with pictures from your clinic. For example, kids, dogs, and team photos score high in positive reactions. If you need inspiration or ideas, check out some of the big brands that are growing fast on Instagram in the beauty space, including Sephora, WunderBrow, and CoverGirl.

Tag People and Brands

When you tag someone in a photo, he or she automatically receives a notification, and the photo is added to his or her "Photos of You" section. This will ensure that the person tagged sees your image, and increases the likelihood that he or she will share the photo with his or her followers and comment on it.

Include Location

Include the location of your photo or video when it helps tell the story of the image. Use the Add People feature to tag accounts in your image when they will help you reach a broader audience. Remember to follow privacy regulations; to be safe, avoid tagging patients.

Post Intro

The intro to a post is important to get right. Do not just post an image without a description or it loses some of its value. Choose story lines that are authentic to your brand and are well conveyed through captivating imagery. Each graphic requires some explanation of what it is, and why Instagrammers should like and share it. Keep it to about three lines on your phone because on Instagram, it is really all about the visual.

Use Relevant Hashtags

The preferred order of posting on Instagram is text, emojis, and then a string of hashtags.

Hashtags are an integral part of Instagram, and posts almost feel naked without them. Many posts include a long chain of hashtags. Keep captions short and pithy. Incorporate a few hashtags but not so many that they detract from the simplicity of the post. Use the same hashtags throughout your social platforms for consistency, and add to your core list as needed.

Hashtags are searchable on Instagram, so they are important in helping people find and follow you, and in regramming (i.e., sharing). You can post additional text or hashtags in a comment below your post, and it will work the same way as your description in terms of searchable text.

Instagram also allows you to edit posts once they go live. Go to the three-dot button on the upper right corner of your post, and click on the drop-down menu that offers the options to Archive, Turn Off Commenting, Edit, Share, or Delete.

HASHTAG EXAMPLES

- Brand or product hashtags (#Botox #Coolsculpting)
- Contest hashtags (if you are running a contest)
- General keyword hashtags (#bodyshaping #skinlaser #skincare #dermatologist #cosmeticsurgeon)
- Event hashtags (#FACE2018 #IMCAS2018)
- Trending hashtags (based on news and pop culture)
- Location-based hashtags (#London #NYC #BeverlyHills)

Another way to engage with other users is to like and comment on their images, and respond to comments or questions on your own posts in a timely manner.

Check for hashtags that have the most users, which indicates that more people are searching for them, but keep them relevant to your text. Use the most important hashtags first, as more hashtags will not get found in searches. Get keyword savvy about what your clinic offers. For example, if your post is about skincare, include #skincare #beautyproducts #skincaretips #beautifulskin, for starters. You can also get creative. Since I travel so much, I will often use the hashtag #OOTD for "office of the day" instead of the more familiar "outfit of the day."

25 RELEVANT INSTAGRAM HASHTAGS

Instagram Hashtags

#Beauty	#Beautyaddict
#Medicalspa	#Skincare
#Cosmeticsurgery	#Beforeandafter
#Plasticsurgeon	#Transformation
#Transformationtuesday	#Instabeauty
#Plasticsurgery	#Results
#Makeover	#Aesthetics
#BeautifulSkin	#Cosmetics
#Antiaging	#Tummytuck
#Dermatologist	#Lipfillers
#Botox	#Healthyskin
#Brazilianbuttlift or #BBL	#Wrinkles
#FatFreeFriday	

Optimize Your Posts

Instagram does not offer the analytics features that Facebook does. Therefore, you will need to get your numbers and results from third parties for now. One good tool is Iconosquare that offers a way to track what is and is not working. You can see most liked and commented on photos and videos, optimal days and frequency to post based on your followers, best performing photo filters, and stats about your followers and who you are following.

Getting Likes and Shares

As on every social platform, to get likes and shares you need to be very active and visible on Instagram. Commenting, regramming, and liking posts from accounts you follow is an essential strategy to build up your profile. The way to cultivate a following is to follow like-minded users and follow back people who follow you and like, comment, and share your posts.

No one is going to see your posts if you do not have followers. Use the free tools to search e-mails and Facebook for current fans you have. Once you have enough fans, start posting images or a 10 second video that relates to your brand. Instagram offers another opportunity for you to build a relationship with your customers. Know your audience to include the right language that they can relate to. Make your clinic brand popular and friendly to give them a reason to continue to follow and engage with you.

Find influencers from the aesthetic industry, colleagues, vendors, brands, and local businesses who are relevant to your brand to follow. If you have separate personal and professional Instagram accounts, consider making the personal one private to block patients from following you. The clinic or business Instagram needs to be public to build a following and promote your brand. *Do not* follow current or past patients.

Ideally, your ratio of followers to people you are following should be substantial. For example, Middle Eastern Instagram makeup artist, blogger, and cosmetics queen Huda (@Hudabeauty) has 20.8 million Instagram followers, yet she is only following 284 accounts as of July 2017. That ratio is not realistic for an aesthetic clinic, however. You need to follow users to get followed back, but once you reach a sufficient ratio, you can start unfollowing users to improve your numbers. Whom you follow makes all the difference, and creating strategic relationships is key. (For example, chances are that Beyoncé and the Duke and Duchess of Cambridge will not follow back.)

Whether your subject is a person or an object, capture it in a context that gives a sense of your point of view. Posting high-quality images or videos daily or every other day may be sufficient to keep it growing. Produce images and videos that feel at home on the platform by editing and using cool filters and other tools. These effects give images that unmistakable "Insta" look that people will respond to. Post photos and videos of beautiful and unexpected moments that will feel authentic and immediate. The more good content you post, the faster you can build up followers.

Instagram Stories

Instagram Stories have quickly surpassed Snapchat as the "go-to" platform for photo and video disappearing content. This allows users to share photos and videos in slideshow format. It is a good idea to separate your followers to test out this strategy and judge responses accordingly. Stories go beyond filter options and can encompass text, drawing, stickers, and other cool features to make these unique to your brand. This plus live broadcasting features make Instagram Stories an ideal vehicle for clinics to take their creativity to a new level by creating attention-grabbing photos and videos. Subjects may include a sneak peek at a new treatment or product, or a behind-the-scenes look at a day in the life of the clinic or a specific practitioner.

Instagram-Sponsored Posts

Ads are a fact of life in the digital world. There are no free rides anymore. Most Instagram users are not exactly fans of the ads that pop up, but they have grown accustomed to them as they have on every other maturing social network. Social media is big business and has overtaken traditional forms of advertising, most notably print. Instagram will notify you if your post is performing better than other content, and suggest promoting it. It takes literally 2 minutes to do so; go to post and click Promote, and you will be prompted to make your selections in terms of what you want to get more of, objective, destination, action button, audience, budget, and duration. You can promote a post for as little as $10.

Influencer Marketing

One strategic way to build your Instagram page is to align your clinic or brand with influencers. Influencers represent a new frontier in marketing—one where brands rely on the popularity of individuals within a specific niche, and then leverage that influencer's relationship with his or her audience to reach their target demographic. They don't have to be celebrities (although that can help). An influencer can be anyone with a strong following and the ability to sway. It should be someone your customers can relate to or that they trust in your industry. They can help you gain a new audience that you may not have otherwise been able to reach. Your goal is also to engage the group of individuals who are already interested in your products and services.

Influencer marketing has sired a cottage industry with firms that specialize in identifying and engaging social media influencers, but your influencers are likely hidden in plain sight. If you really want to find out who influences your patients, just ask them. They will point you to sources that actually make an impact on their decisions. What blogs are on their must-read lists? Whose Instagram pages do they eat up? Instagram is the top platform for brands and companies to hunt for influencers.

A large following alone does not always an influencer make. Followers can be bought; long-term engagement cannot. Once you have developed a list of potential influencers, take a deeper dive into their level of engagement, their organic mentions in social media (other fans and followers talking about the influencer), and their standing with like-minded individuals of importance to your target audience.

People who post a lot of content that is obviously sponsored risk losing their credibility quickly. Be careful to choose someone who is selective about whom he or she partners with and discloses their affiliations in accordance with Federal Trade Commission (FTC) or other relevant regulations.

Reaching Out

Do not start off by contacting influencers offers to "partner with them." Instead, flirt a little. Take small steps to make your presence known. Once you have your whittled-down list, engage with each on their social media and blog posts. Make comments, ask questions, and try to contribute to the conversation. Notice who responds and who does not.

As you build up relationships with potential influencer candidates, ask them to review your product or try a complimentary treatment, and even create content for you. Compensate your influencers by acknowledging them, promoting their work, sharing links and tagging them, or offering treatments and discounts, but most influencers today expect to be compensated the old-fashioned way—with cold, hard cash.

There is no financial baseline to follow, or any standards for fees influencers charge. For example, a C-list Kardashian (not KKW) may charge $100,000+ for a single post, while one of the Housewives of (fill in blank) may ask for $25,000. Once the agents, handlers, and lawyers get involved, they need to get their 15% off the top, too. A local beauty blogger may be happy with a lip filler treatment to write about her experience in your clinic, which may be more impactful to your brand.

THE RISE OF MICROINFLUENCERS

We are not only focused on glitzy celebrities anymore; influencers can be anyone with a following who has the clout to amplify his or her message and influence an audience. It can take just one person sharing a piece of content for the right brand or individual to amplify it significantly. Everyone has access to some channel or platform that could get their content into the hands of people who matter, from soccer moms to socialites.

When you work with an influencer, start by making a list of "asks" to arrive at an arrangement that works for both of you. This may include a blog post, three tweets, a Facebook post, Instagram stories, Snapchat stories, video for YouTube, and so on. You may use influencers to run sponsored posts on their accounts to amplify their reach. It is best to let the influencers post on their channels to expose your brand to their fans and followers, which will be greater than your clinic's network.

Where possible, try to develop a personal relationship with the influencers you have identified on your own, and work out an agreement that seems fair to both parties, with clearly defined parameters to avoid potential misunderstandings. You don't want to enter into a relationship that goes south, especially with someone who has 50,000 fans to trash you to. Return on investment (ROI) can be measured by assigning unique trackable URLs for each influencer, or supplying them with promo codes. This will let you know who is swaying and who is playing.

Betting on the right influencers can elevate your profile to the next level and put you on the map. But this is a double-edged sword and needs to be managed carefully.

FOLLOW THE RULES

Organizations like the U.S. Federal Trade Commission (FTC) and the UK's Advertising Standards Association (ASA) monitor the use of influencers, and they are regulated in several ways. For example, they are not permitted to officially talk about an experience with a product if they have not tried it. If an influencer was paid to try a product and thought it was terrible, the influencer cannot say it is amazing. Influencers also cannot make claims about a product that would require proof the advertiser does not have. Some influencers use hashtags like "#spon" or "#ad" in posts to denote all or some of the above. In most cases, the preferred language would be the word "sponsored" rather than shortening it so it becomes unrecognizable, as in "sp." Legal departments in bigger brands as well as social platforms are also cracking down on the blatant misrepresentation of some influencers as it concerns promoting products and brands to consumers. This practice has become a big issue in social media marketing circles. In response, social platforms are making it harder and harder to skirt around this rule. Facebook and Instagram are launching new tools that require an influencer to list the brand as a business partner on a piece of sponsored content. Watch this space!

Twitter: Promoting Your Clinic in 280 Characters

Twitter is an entirely mobile form of communication, largely because the posts are only 280 characters as of November 2017, and therefore simpler to do on the go: users can tweet through their computers, tablets, or mobile phones from anywhere.

The advantages Twitter offers include brevity (280 characters) and immediacy (users communicate in real time). This can be beneficial for the dissemination of time-sensitive news. Once something is tweeted and retweeted by another user, it is forever in the public domain and cannot be retracted.

Due to the current state of the world, Twitter has become a hotbed of controversy. Steer clear of politics and religion. If you have interesting content, Twitter is a great tool for quickly spreading the word. Retweeting and sharing other users' content is quite simple, and if a user with a lot of followers retweets you, your content has the potential to be seen by a lot of additional users.

To attract followers, it is essential to share interesting, relevant content from other Twitter users to keep your followers engaged and interested.

To build a meaningful base of followers, focus on these categories:

* Content
* Engagement
* Rewards

Good content is readily shareable. It should be compelling and quality information that is of interest to your followers. Engagement can be nurtured with your audience by asking questions, engaging in debate and dialogue, and even asking for retweets. Rewards can also be offered by way of social-media-only deals (last-minute appointments or treatment courses, gift with purchase) or by posting behind-the-scenes images of the clinic that are exclusive to your followers.

If you don't want to spend a lot of time on Twitter, consider automating specific posts. I prefer automating Facebook to Twitter, but *never* go from Twitter to Facebook. Note that this is not considered best practice, but it is a huge time saver for busy clinics without a social media team in place.

The idea of a doctor tweeting while he is doing a laser treatment or a facelift, can demedicalize what you do. Maintain your professionalism online.

The microblogging platform is also a place for people to connect with brands and is often considered the new customer relationship management tool. Twitter has also emerged as a strong leader among social media platforms in terms of stimulating conversations about current events, pop culture, and brands. Users turn to Twitter when looking to speak directly to a brand or find out about others' experience with a brand.

Practitioners can use Twitter to announce news and events and to promote special offers, events, and media appearances. It also drives followers to your website, Facebook page, YouTube channel, and blog when linked back to these sources. Twitter is a great way to engage with bloggers, media, and other influencers, as well as leverage any media appearances you may participate in.

Think of it as a virtual word-of-mouth platform that allows users to share their immediate thoughts on people and places. For aesthetic practitioners, engaging via Twitter can allow positive impressions to be built and shared and brand ambassadors to be developed. By prompting users to retweet your tweets and share their favorable opinions with their followers, it can lead to an increase in traffic and revenue.

From Tweeting to Treating

Twitter options for customization allow you to brand your Twitter account easily. The best strategy is to link your Twitter to your Facebook page so that posts are automatically shared with Twitter. Thus, if you are not ready to dedicate a lot of time to tweeting, Facebook posts will serve as content to at least keep it going until you can focus on this channel more seriously.

Create a profile with information about your clinic and brand. Strive to build your following, reputation, and customer trust through sharing photos and "behind the scenes" glimpses of your practice (i.e., special promotion for Twitter followers). Assign someone to monitor comments that users post about your clinic, brand, and practitioners.

Choose your Twitter account name wisely; for example, many practices have one account for the practice, and one for the individual physician(s): @johnsonaesthetic and @drjohnjohnson. You can use a maximum of 15 characters for your username, and it can be changed any time.

Add a Header Photo

You can change your profile and header photos any time:

- Photos can be in JPG, GIF, or PNG formats
- Dimensions for profile photos are 400×400 pixels
- Dimensions for header photos are 1500×500 pixels

Navigating Twitter

On the right of your home page will be a stream of tweets posted by the people you follow. The more people you follow, the more interesting this page becomes. To tweet, click the top right corner of your page. You can link to images, videos, or web URLs and add a location if you want to show users where you are. A tweet allows up to 280 characters, but it is recommended to leave space for retweets and comments.

BREAKING NEWS: Links or URLs to images and videos are no longer included in the 280-character limit (which are calculated as letters including spaces).

Your Interactions timeline shows you how others have been interacting with you on Twitter. Twitter will notify you when someone marks your tweet as a favorite, mentions your username, follows you, or retweets (shares) your content. When another user includes your username preceded by the @ symbol in a tweet, that is a "Mention."

Start Tweeting

Build your voice. Retweet, reply, and react. Show users what you care about and what you are following. Retweet messages you like or reply to a tweet by using the @ symbol and their username. Mention others in your content by their Twitter username (preceded by @) in your tweets. This can help draw more eyes to your message and start new conversations.

Using Hashtags

People use the hashtag symbol # with no spaces before a relevant keyword or phrase in their tweet to categorize those tweets and show up in a Twitter search. Clicking on a hashtagged word in any message shows you all other tweets marked with that keyword and can appear anywhere in the tweet. Hashtagged words that are trending will be listed in "Trending Topics."

Example of hashtagged tweet: *#Laserresurfacing now avail at Dr. Smith's Aesthetics Clinic Surrey! #freeconsultation bit.ly/smithaesthetics.com*

If you tweet with a hashtag on a public (not private) account, anyone who does a search for that hashtag can find your tweet.

To Delete a Tweet

You can only delete tweets sent from your account. Locate the tweet you want to delete. Hover your mouse over the message—Done! If it has already been retweeted after you posted it, you cannot retract it, and it could get retweeted again and again indefinitely.

Retweeting Others' Content

Twitter's retweet feature helps you and others quickly share a tweet with all of your followers. Users may type RT at the beginning of a tweet to indicate that they are reposting someone else's content.

Example of a retweet: *#RT @Wendylewisco Just had my brown spots lasered away with the newest fractionated system #NYCPlasticsurgeon @drbryangforley #nopain*

Twitter Ads

To advertise on Twitter, go to business.twitter.com/. Twitter offers a sophisticated self-service platform—Twitter Ads Manager—to help you create campaigns, promote brand awareness, and gain new followers. But your campaigns will only be as successful as the quality of tweets you create to promote, and users are much more likely to engage with tweets containing visuals, images, and video.

Targeted campaigns offer four options for goals:

- Get website traffic
- Grow Twitter followers
- Promote brand awareness
- Increase engagement

Promoted tweets help to reach a wider audience or to spark engagement from your followers. They are clearly labeled "Promoted" to denote that you have paid for their placement. These tweets can be retweeted, replied to, favorited, and more.

You can target by "Location," "Language," "Age," "Gender," "Relationship status," "Interested in," and "Education" on Facebook, and "Country(s)" on Twitter. If you want to send out a post to people who speak Spanish, geo-targeting is an easy way to do it.

Twitter allows businesses to locate their current customers or seek out potential customers. For example, if you open a medspa in the neighborhood, you can create a geo search to identify anyone tweeting about beauty, skin, makeup, and so on, within your area. After locating those individuals, start reaching out to invite them to come try a treatment and experience your medspa.

Another handy feature for the time-deprived marketer is Quick Promote (business.twitter.com/en/advertising/campaign-types/quick-promote.html). This tool gets your tweets seen by more users for better engagement. It is ideal to use from your phone, and to promote events and speaking engagements by live tweeting on the fly.

If you are serious about using Twitter to market your clinic, an ad strategy is essential for success. Start small, track your analytics, and add to the budget when you see results on a tweet-by-tweet basis. Test multiple ads to see which perform best for your clinic. Check out how much you are paying per new follower or increased engagement, and determine if it is worth that amount to your brand.

9

Photo Sharing Platforms

Photography takes an instant out of time, altering life by holding it still.

Dorothea Lange

Content that includes an image is far more appealing and, thus, will achieve more impressions, shares, likes, and comments. Numerous studies have shown that a social media post with an image or other visual gets far more engagement compared to a post with only words and no image or link. Even tweets with images have been shown to get much higher rates of retweets.

Personal images are clearly the best route to take, such as photos of the clinic, staff, your community, a cake baked by a patient, flowers sent as a thank you gesture, the doctor in action or at a speaking engagement, and so on. These communicate more personally with your fans and followers.

If you are taking photos of people, make them "happy snaps" that show actual faces, use their names if possible, and capture their eyes and smiles. Photos of people engaging with each other also work nicely.

Tagging your brand's photo assets helps you sort through your own images faster, as well as help make them easily discoverable for other users. If your goal for photo sharing is to engage your social media audience and join the ongoing conversation, use tags. If you are keen to take photos of events to share on social media, go with a network that allows you to tag other users in the photos, such as Instagram. If you are more interested in engaging with local users, take advantage of geo-tagging options on key platforms.

Photo Editing Hacks

If you do not have a dedicated graphic design team, you will benefit from photo editing hacks in the form of apps and filters. Consistent, high-quality visual media can boost audience engagement and reinforce your brand's high standards. Different networks offer a varying degree of complexity in editing: Instagram allows users to apply filters for basic editing in the app, like cropping, adding highlights, or adding a vignette.

For the most part, you will need to go to the Apple Store or Google Play and search through the wide variety of editing apps and filters that can take your images and video to the next level.

Search under these categories:

- Design
- Graphics
- Photo editor
- Photography
- Social media
- Social networking
- Video

Look for apps that have four- to five-star ratings, and read the top comments to decide if they are worth it. Under "Photography apps," for example, there are 1,982 choices to date, and this number increases constantly. Also check the right column under "Apps for photographers" and "Apps for designers." Most apps are free to download and use a basic version with what is called "in-app purchases." Most are very affordable. Some of these are platform specific, while others can enhance your own photos with filters and clever add-ons to make your visuals get noticed.

APPS THAT WILL CHANGE YOUR LIFE

App	Description	Cost
Boomerang	Video app—capture short moments to relive in a loop	Free
Hyperlapse	Create stunning time-lapse videos	Free
Layout	Create fun layouts by remixing your own photos	Free
Mextures	Apply film grain, textures, light leaks, and beautiful gradients for images	$1.99
Hipstamatic	Shoot beautiful authentic photography	$2.99
Repost	#Repost your favorite photos and videos on Instagram while giving the credit to the original Instagrammer	Free
Pic Stitch	Quickly combine multiple pics or videos into one beautifully framed photo	In-app purchases
Word Swag	Turn your words into beautiful text designs or caption your photos	Free/In-app purchases
Giphy	Finding the perfect GIF could not be easier	Free
Rhonna Designs	Cool fonts, frames, and designs for your photos	$1.99
YouCam Perfect	Make every pic perfect with the best selfie camera and photo editing app	$1.99
Photo Plastic	Reshape and simulate realistic plastic surgeries	$0.99
Facetune	For taking great selfies on your iPhone	Free
MakeupPlus	Take your selfie editing to the next level	Free
ImgPlay	Make GIFs or videos using live photos, burst photos, and video	$1.99
Ripl	Custom animated posts for Facebook, Instagram, Twitter	In-app purchases
Instagram In-App Filters	Gingham, Moon, Aden, Hudson, Earlybird, Vesper, Stinson, Charmes	Free
	Iconosquare	In-app purchases

Pinterest Strategy

WARNING: Pinterest is highly addictive. Proceed with caution.

Pinterest is a platform that features digital bulletin boards where users can save and display content they like in the form of pins. You create and organize boards by category, so for example, you might start with a board dedicated to skincare where you would pin the following: *Our Favorite Eye Creams, Top Acne Tips, Best UV Protection*, and so on.

At its most basic, Pinterest is a format for spreading joy and sharing inspiration. The concept is simple; you see something that strikes your fancy, you like it, and you pin it, so that your network of followers can enjoy it, too. While it may seem that Pinterest has a casual, friendly, and social feel to it, do not lose sight of the opportunity to create boards and add pins that have to do with your practice and the services you offer. Social consumption sites such as Pinterest are excellent marketing avenues for consumer products. Businesses establish presences on these platforms and use the unique properties of each to highlight who they are and what they do. Individuals can like or follow businesses they are interested in.

The good news for aesthetic clinics, cosmetic surgeons, and dermatologists is that Pinterest skews heavily female. Women are engaging on Pinterest much more than men in general, which is true of most social platforms. The very nature of Pinterest as an aggregate board of everyone's pins allows users to follow friends' interests, which tends to resonate with a female mind-set. So, if you are operating on, injecting, or lasering women, or selling skincare, you should consider checking out Pinterest. It is extremely time consuming, so the last thing you want to do is have your receptionist, who should be answering the phone and taking care of patients to pay the bills, pinning in the middle of the day.

Think of Pinterest as complementary to your main social media channels and consider posting when you have good content to share that suits your online message. Pinterest is very visual; every post has to be an image or video. Keeping pin boards organized and search-friendly by adding hashtags takes some creativity. "Pinning" allows its users to share and curate ideas by pinning images or videos to their pinboards. Users and fellow pinners can then choose to follow your boards on various consumer-friendly topics, such as body shaping, skin resurfacing, or acne skincare, for example.

Pinterest can engage consumers with images of your practice, including products and treatments, and offer up a more personal look at the doctors, staff, and mission. For example, you can create a Medical Team board and include a photo and bio for each person, and feature photos of events you have participated in, or the doctor's personal picks for skincare products. Pinterest skews largely female, and many mothers and grandmothers, and therefore users, are very interested in knowing interesting and unique insider facts. It is like being a member in a private club, and the content should take on a more personal and entertaining tone than other platforms.

Pinterest can increase visibility among the audiences that matter and driving traffic to your website and other social networks. It is the network of choice for shopaholics and people who like to plan holidays, weddings, events, and parties, as well as travel, decorating, crafts, and design. Pinterest is also a powerful driver to popular e-commerce sites like Shopify, Etsy, Amazon, and eBay.

Join Pinterest as a Business

Business pages offer additional features, benefits, and analytics that personal pages don't offer, so it is well worthwhile. If you already have a personal page, you can convert it to a business page in a few clicks. Pinterest analytics can help you learn what and when to pin to get the most traction. Like all social platforms, even if you do not yet plan to get active on Pinterest, at least join as a business and reserve your name for the future.

You can use up to 200 characters to describe your clinic in the About section. Add some keywords or phrases based on Google Analytics to see what drives people to your website. Add a description to take advantage of search engine optimization on Pinterest that is clear and to the point. Include links back to your website or blog.

Try to reserve content exclusively for Pinterest that is not used in the same way on other platforms. Facebook and Twitter content does not really perform well on Pinterest; there is an inherent difference in the user experience and desired formats. Search for relevant businesses, organizations, media, and colleagues to connect with them on Pinterest. Pinterest offers many options for content creation, including videos, slide shows, and podcasts, in addition to images of all kinds.

Pinterest Best Practices

Like Instagram, the most attractive and visually appealing images get liked and repinned the most. For example, infographics and beautiful photography from magazines rate high. The strategy of charting the history of a brand, product, or treatment through an archive of images is also popular.

Pinterest is not a platform where purely self-promotional content will go far. To use Pinterest for your clinic, start pinning from various sources rather than just your own site. Pinning from within Pinterest is the best way to engage with other users and build a robust network. Use descriptions of your pins strategically to increase optimization. You want to ensure that your pins are findable, and include a reference link back to your website to drive traffic where relevant, without overdoing it.

To make sure your boards and pins look appealing, pay attention to the size of your images. Long, skinny pins tend to be the most clicked-on image sizes because they require you to click on them so you can see the full size to read. Pinterest forces you to think more visually.

Pinterest is about celebration and inspiration. Eyes, lips, nails, and legs are popular. Fashion is always good. Ditto for celebrity content. You should add a caption on every pin that you post so that it is more recognizable and relatable to your brand. Inspiration on Pinterest comes in many forms, with pins that share quotes, art, movies, books, actors, celebs, special events, and more. Quotes are a particularly rich source of repins. Travel images of great places are also good. Create your own inspirational pins by using famous quotes or creating your own, and add your logo to make them uniquely yours. Continually pinning, repinning, following, and refreshing pinboards is important to keep your followers engaged.

Creating Boards

Get started on Pinterest by creating boards. Boards are the cornerstone of the Pinterest platform, and you can create as many as you like, and be as specific as you want to be. Of the boards found in search results for "Pinterest for business," those that appear on the top of the list include keywords directly in the board name. Strive to make your boards more findable. Use boards to reflect the issues that are in line with your brand and to stay visible and interesting to your followers. As you plan new Pinterest boards, consider how seasons, holidays, and events dovetail with your social media calendar. Pinterest boards will be more discoverable via search when the board name contains keywords. Consider creating boards for holidays, seasons, and general beauty themes that are relevant to your target audiences. Pinboard traffic is affected by seasons and holidays. Seasonal boards can be updated each year and relocated to the bottom of your profile page as you add content to them when you run across it.

Designate Boards for Aspects of Your Practice

Curate boards that share information of interest to your target audience, as well as boards that relate to your practice. Create at least a few boards that cover a broad range of interests, rather than maintaining a single board devoted to one topic (like laser resurfacing or rhinoplasty) or your practice alone.

Start with a handful of themes and add boards aligned with them, and pin images that are visually attractive and aligned with the theme. For example, show users where you are and how they can find you with visuals. Include a board for a charity you may be active in, or an event that your clinic is participating in. Include boards that are not entirely related to your practice so as to open engagement with a wider range of audiences.

To collaborate with influencers, colleagues, or partners on Pinterest, create a group board and invite users to pin to your board. Your invitees can contribute to the board, but as the creator, you will be the only person able to change the title and description. You can also remove pinners and any inappropriate pins from the board.

12 IDEAS FOR PINTEREST BOARDS

- Holidays
- Seasons
- Inspirational quotes
- Cosmetics
- Skincare tips
- Body shaping
- Anti-aging
- Beauty tutorials
- Bridal beauty

- Famous people
- Celebrities
- Eco-friendly beauty

The goal of engagement on Pinterest is to get repinned or shared; it is not just about followers.

Make sure your website images are found when users are searching the web for pins. Name your images with keywords so they are search engine friendly, and incorporate hashtags into your pins for increased visibility.

Use Pinterest to identify influencers who already have the attention of your target audience. Start by following them and repinning the content you like. Like their pins and make comments to start a dialogue. As with most social platforms, liking someone's pins will encourage them to like you back. Engaging with other commenters is an important aspect of Pinterest. Make sure your social media community managers respond to the comments and questions users post on pins. Take the time to share meaningful comments on influencers' boards.

Exploring Rich Pins

Pinterest has five types of rich pins that let you add topic-specific details to a pin:

1. Article pins include the headline, author, story description, and link.
2. Product pins include real-time pricing, availability, and where to buy.
3. Recipe pins include ingredients, cooking times, and serving info.
4. Movie pins include ratings, cast members, and reviews.
5. Place pins include an address, phone number, and map.

Decide which you want to apply for, add the appropriate metatags to your site, and validate your rich pins. Use rich pins to give users more relevant information about the pins that interest them. Use rich pins in moderation for key content to get more engagement.

What Not to Do

Do not create boards named Rhytidectomy, Blepharoplasty, Fractional Lasers, and so on. Choose consumer-friendly health and beauty themes. Before and after photos of a 65-year-old woman who had a neck lift will not perform well on Pinterest. However, an after picture of an attractive patient who had a great result is appropriate. Avoid anything too clinical, bloody, or graphic. A picture of a laser is also not visually interesting. This is the polar opposite of what Pinterest is all about.

Pinterest Ads

Pinterest offers some good options for promoting your pins in the form of Promoted Pins that you pay for to get your content seen by more users. Pinterest ads can be very affordable and help generate traction for your boards.

Pinterest offers three types of ad campaigns:

- **Awareness campaigns**—These aim to get you noticed by pinners who do not already know you. You pay per 1,000 impressions.
- **Engagement campaigns**—These are designed to encourage pinners to interact with your content by repinning or clicking on your Promoted Pins. You pay per engagement action.

- **Traffic campaigns**—These are used to send people from your Pinterest ads directly to your website. You Pay Per Click.

The process is the same for creating all three types of Promoted Pins, so dive in and get started on your first Pinterest ad campaign.

All social platforms now require some level of investment in the form of ads and promoted content to be seen and deliver results. You work hard, curate content, create graphics, write copy, and nothing happens. It is frustrating and demoralizing. Without some paid boosts, your efforts will not deliver sufficiently measurable results, which accounts for the drop-off rates on social media. It is common to get frustrated at stalled engagement or limited follower counts, but I promise you there will be rewards longterm for those who stick it out. Don't give up!

10

The Value of Video

Video is the most interesting and engaging way to share an idea with others.

Chad Hurley

Video marketing is trending. This is one of the key strategies you should get on board with quickly. Prospective patients want to feel like they know you before they ever come to your clinic, and current patients also enjoy seeing videos of their aesthetic practitioners online to stay connected with your brand.

Creating videos of some of the interesting things you do every day can be a very effective component of a clinic marketing plan. Consumers relate well to content that is visually appealing, well thought out, eye catching, and has a personal touch.

Snapchat offers less filtered, more immediate glimpses into daily life as well as scripted events. And just as with real life, the videos are short lived, lasting from 10 seconds to 24 hours, which encourages people to participate in real time. These new social media platforms are changing the landscape of behind-the-scenes access, offering unfiltered views of everything from megawatt award shows to a glimpse of what goes on in your office.

It is a brave new world.

Best Video Formats

The first video to consider creating for your marketing program is a 2–3 minute video clip that lives on the landing page of your clinic website. I refer to it as a "Welcome to my practice" theme. Patients cannot get a sense of who you are from a still photograph anymore, especially at low resolution on a mobile device. Therefore, placing a short and sweet video on your website can draw patients in to get a sense of their comfort level with you as a practitioner.

It is a good idea to write out a script or at least bullet points to guide you through the recording, although you can improvise along the way to avoid seeming like you are reading from a teleprompter. The most sincere video clips are on topics the subject knows well and is passionate about. You should appear to be relaxed and comfortable. Record a few variations to schedule them at specific intervals in the future. Depending on your appetite for more, videos of the consultation process and treatment demonstrations are also great to have in your marketing armamentarium.

If you are planning to promote your clinic with a new or unique treatment, having *b-roll* of the practitioner performing the treatment is also nice to have on hand. B-roll is footage that television networks typically use as a cutaway to help tell the story. It can be used to introduce a segment or between interviews in the background. Generally, no sound is used, which allows for voice-over or music to be added as needed. Television stations will sometimes ask for b-roll when considering if a pitch idea is media worthy. This footage can also be used in other ways, such as on YouTube, Facebook, your website, and other social platforms.

Keep in mind that your video-recording area should be good quality, with consistent lighting and background. You can use a backdrop or a bare wall if you prefer, although sitting at your desk may be more natural and comfortable for you. Dress for your target audience—clean scrubs, a white coat, or a suit jacket as appropriate. If you are not comfortable in front of the camera, enlist a professional videographer. Record several takes to make sure you get the best possible sound bites and quality, and eliminate any background noise like traffic, music, doorbells, phones, or footsteps that may arise.

This process is a skill worth mastering. You may choose to run your recorded material through an editing program, which can greatly improve the professionalism of your videos, or have an experienced videographer help you with editing. Titles, credits, background music, and simple special effects can be added with video creating/editing software, if desired.

10 GREAT IDEAS FOR VIDEO SNIPPETS

- Consultations with patients with signed consent
- Nonsurgical treatments—injections, lasers, light therapy, etc.
- Surgical procedures—preferably with patients' private areas carefully draped
- Aestheticians performing spa therapies
- Hair restoration procedures
- Real patients talking about their experiences
- Introduction to staff members
- Staff having treatments
- Patients' friends/family talking about their experience
- Tour of the clinic facility

Patient Videos

One of the most common video themes used is the "Patient Diary" or "Patient Journey" style. These can be extremely compelling videos showing the patient from consultation through recovery and final result, or any variation on that theme. This tactic is especially helpful when the procedure being documented is one that can have a healing process that could turn patients off. Seeing how another patient fares can overcome those objections and make the patient feel more comfortable going ahead with the procedure.

Testimonials are the new word of mouth. As clinics are so concerned about reviews and ratings, videos from real patients talking about their experience are extremely compelling. It is common to see handwritten notes and e-mails with the patient's name blacked out posted on websites. That is fine, too, but video is more compelling. Because we know the importance of what other patients are saying about your clinic and the work you do, this is a great way to counterbalance online reviews. These should be from legitimate real patients, not staff or family. It must ring true to viewers. Real people want to hear from other real people who are relatable and sincere.

Whatever you post should mirror the target audience you are going after. A patient doing the talking is word of mouth at its best. Used in the right way, testimonials can influence potential patients to choose you over your competition. In fact, when it comes to medical practice marketing, testimonials are essential, because they are evidence of your ability as a practitioner and they provide prospective customers with an expectation for results. When a prospective patient identifies with a patient who has given a testimonial, it helps the prospective patient understand more about the solutions you offer and how they relate to her. Testimonials also give you instant credibility. People are always more comfortable when they see a real person, with real results, and an honest opinion endorse your practice.

Testimonials have taken on new meaning in the age of online reviews. A website overflowing with testimonials from happy patients sharing their experiences is a compelling clinic building tool. It works because the testimonials reaffirm for potential clients that your aesthetic practice stands out and serve to validate an image of excellence with a message that is distinctly authentic. This form of communication can greatly influence purchasing decisions. Savvy consumers are seeking independent confirmation in the form of sincere endorsements from actual customers.

NOTE: If the patient decides she does not want the video on your site, social channels, or YouTube at any time in the future, the patient has the right to ask for it to be taken down.

6 TIPS FOR GREAT TESTIMONIALS

1. Reach out to patients who are most like your key target audience.
2. Make sure they have a compelling and positive story to tell about their experiences in your practice.
3. Choose patients whose stories will highlight the key aspects of your practice, such as popular procedures, treatments, and aftercare services.
4. Always say "thank you" when patients agree to give you a testimonial; make sure they know how much you appreciate their support. Rewarding a patient after the testimonial is done is fine, but incentivizing patients to write positive reviews in advance is frowned upon.
5. Gather a robust selection of testimonials in different formats: personal thank you notes, letters, e-mails, comments given by phone or to staff members, and video. If a patient gives you a gift of flowers or sweets, highlight this on social media by posting, "We have the best patients!" (No name required)
6. Get testimonials about new procedures you have added to the practice, and those you want to highlight, such as a new fat melting system or a signature facelift technique.

How to Ask for Testimonials

WENDYISM

The best advertisement for an aesthetic practitioner is a happy patient who is willing to talk about the experience.

Some patients will volunteer to give you an endorsement. When this happens, ask them to write their testimonials in their own words quickly before they forget. For patients who are pleased with your products and services but don't offer to provide you with a testimonial, you must simply ask. Patients who are truly pleased with your clinic and work may be inclined to give you a testimonial, but you must *ask* for it. A testimonial is best taken when the patient comes in for a follow-up visit, since they may not recall the experience after an extended period of time.

Think about any recent e-mails you have received from patients to say thanks. Maybe you received positive feedback from someone who responded to a survey you sent out. When a client says great things about you, your work, or your staff, give the client the opportunity to turn that praise into a testimonial. Say something like this, "We would really appreciate it if we can include what you just said in our testimonials. Would that be okay with you?" If a patient says something like, "This has been a great experience and I am so glad I chose you," respond by asking if she would mind giving you a testimonial for your website or writing a review on a forum that is relevant to your practice. You may be pleasantly surprised at how many patients may be willing to do it for you.

Make a list of potential contacts to approach. Depending on your relationship, this can be done by phone, e-mail, or when they come in for a visit. If the patient is particularly fond of a staff member, it may be best left to them. Ask if the patient would allow his or her first and/or last names to be used, initials, age, location, and photos. In most cases, patients will want to be anonymous, such as "Jill from Northern California," or "J.T., age 56." Never exert pressure or make the patient feel uncomfortable.

You may tactfully ask individuals who have clout with your target market or name recognition if they are willing to use their real names and/or photos. This must be handled delicately. There is tremendous value to your practice to be able to use a local celebrity, TV personality, or beauty queen in your practice materials, but that usually comes at a price.

To get testimonials, make the process as easy as possible for patients. Most people are not comfortable putting words on paper or expressing themselves on camera. The best testimonials do not have to be professional; their value lies in the authenticity. Ask them to answer one key question that gets right to the point, such as "What do you like most about our practice and why?" or "What impact has the treatment you have had with us had on your life?"

Editing Counts

Ideally, allow patients to describe their problems briefly, then let them talk about how they *felt* about the treatment you provided, and then let them brag about the results. Allow patients providing you with testimonials to write or tell you about the experience naturally. You do not want to tell patients what to say, but you can help them shape their testimonials by asking the right questions.

The key to great testimonials lies in flawless editing. Go over the content recorded, and zoom in on the pertinent points. The more personal, the more engaging it will sound. Draft a summary or concise version you want to use, and include direct quotes whenever you can. Share your edited version with the patient before posting it anywhere to be sure he or she is happy with the way it reads or sounds. Once you obtain the patient's approval and signed consent form, your testimonial can go live.

---

5 PROMPTS FOR A VIDEO OR AUDIO TESTIMONIAL

1. What was your experience like in our practice?
2. Ask if they were was initially skeptical about having a treatment done. What were some of the patient's concerns and how was he or she made to feel more comfortable? (I was afraid of going under anesthesia, but the medical staff made me feel very safe, etc.)
3. What specific results did they get from the treatment or procedure they had done? The more details they can add, the better. (I look better than I did at my wedding; I look less tired, etc.)
4. What was the reaction from family, friends, and colleagues? (My husband loves the way I look; my mother wants to have something done now too, etc.)
5. How do you feel after having the procedure? Let them talk about their feelings, not only the results. (I feel so much more confident when I look in the mirror, I love wearing makeup again now that I can see my eyelids, etc.)

All of the above results are proof of the value of the services you offer and will hopefully convey a sense of caring and credibility to prospective patients.

Using Testimonials

Post testimonials where prospective clients are most likely to read them, such as on your website, blog, Facebook page, e-blasts, or in printed promotional materials such as brochures and banners. Create a dedicated page devoted to testimonials, or add them on specific pages related to procedures. Another option is to include quotes from satisfied patients rotating on the landing page.

Testimonials can take many forms. You can repurpose a testimonial into a short quote for your site or use it in an e-book or article for a consumer publication or website. Review your testimonials to refresh them as you gather new ones. Try to post the most recent testimonials in chronological order, with the most recent first. This should be an ongoing process.

Thank patients appropriately for their kind comments about your practice. A handwritten note, flowers, or a call shows appreciation. If you want to be generous, offer the patient a complimentary product, service or treatment, but only AFTER the testimonial is completed. Do not incentivize patients to provide testimonials, as that practice may be considered questionable or unethical in most markets.

Using testimonials to market your clinic is an impactful strategy. In fact, not having patients sing your praises leaves you at a distinct disadvantage.

YouTube Strategy

YouTube, owned by Google, is the social destination for all things video and boasts over one billion users worldwide and four billion daily views.

The global influence of YouTube is off the charts. It is the premier destination to go for video content of all kinds. There is content covering all aspects of health and well-being, treatment videos, surgical footage, and more. The visual nature of this video-sharing site has proven to be a natural fit for aesthetic physicians. Video is ideal for illustrating aesthetic procedures and to help patients get acquainted with your practice. It is also a super popular channel for all your patient targets, from millennials to boomers, both male and female.

YouTube allows you to create a branded channel where you can upload videos that you own the copyright for. Users can subscribe to your channel to view your videos, comment, and like or dislike your posts. They can get notified any time you upload a new video to YouTube, which can keep them coming back. Add a cover photo to customize your channel.

YouTube can be a great forum for people to connect, inform, and inspire other users on any topic you can think of. Video content, along with photos, has emerged as the primary content that gets liked and shared on social media platforms.

YouTube allows users to

- Browse millions of videos uploaded by community members
- Upload, "tag," and share videos worldwide
- Make uploaded videos public
- Find, join, and create groups to connect with people with similar interests
- Subscribe to member videos, save favorites, and create playlists
- Embed YouTube videos into websites with a video embed code

When you upload a video to YouTube, it stays online until you choose to take it down. YouTube may also take it offline if they believe your video violates their terms of use (e.g., adult content or copyright infringement).

Your Clinic Channel

To get started on YouTube, set up a branded channel for your practice. By creating a channel, you will have a public profile and be able to comment, save videos to playlists, and more. Without creating a channel, you can only subscribe and like videos.

The video camera on your iPhone is sufficient quality for this purpose. YouTube only allows you to post original videos or ones you have the rights or permission to use, which does not usually include clips from television appearances. For example, if you were on a national television show, you may be restricted from posting the video clip on YouTube or may require permission or need to pay a fee for the privilege. In that case, you may get away with using a screenshot or clip, but you can certainly post the link on all your marketing platforms.

YouTube can be formatted to allow all new videos added to be posted on Twitter automatically. YouTube encourages you to connect your YouTube channel with a Google+ profile or page to access new features. Most active YouTube channels are already connected to Google+ channel. Users then subscribe to your channel to watch your videos. When you subscribe to relevant channels, their content will show up in your feed.

To post videos, go to the upper right corner of your channel and click Upload. Add the title of the video, add a description, choose the category it should be in, and add tags.

How to optimize your YouTube channel:

- Add a description to your video so that viewers can learn more information about it, which will display at the bottom of the video.
- Tags allow YouTube users to see your video by linking common words associated with your video of "Wrinkle Treatment," "Wrinkle," and "treatment." Other videos with similar tags will be seen in the "Recommended videos" sidebar.
- Annotations allow you to add notes or pauses to the video that you may have overlooked. These allow the viewer to see additional information about your channel without having to read the description.
- Give the video a description that is different than the assigned title.
- To get the most views, keep the title simple, add relevant tags, and include your username as a tag.
- To share your video on a website or social platform, embed it by copying the code YouTube provides.

Creating Videos

Original video content is required on YouTube, which means that you cannot really recycle content easily. But the content does not have to be professional quality. Another option is to hire a videographer who could spend a day or half a day at your clinic making videos of the staff, patients who have consented, procedures being done, or a consultation taking place. One video is not going to be cost effective, but to do five or ten short videos in one day can be worth the spend. The trick is in the editing process, which requires some level of skill.

Video editing apps abound and can be very useful to create more professional videos for your marketing efforts (see page 92 for best video apps).

TrueView Video Ads

YouTube offers a cost-effective video ad program, TrueView, that starts at just $10 per day for a local campaign. The platform offers step-by-step instructions on how to create various types of video ads to promote your practice. Much like other online advertising solutions, you only pay if a user watches your ad for 30 seconds, watches your entire ad, or clicks on your ad. You can create ads to drive viewers to your website or YouTube channel. With TrueView ads, you are only charged when viewers watch or interact with elements of your video. There are two types of TrueView ads: in-stream and video discovery. A big selling point for YouTube's ad platform is that viewers who complete a TrueView ad are more likely to visit or subscribe to a brand channel, watch more from the brand, or share the video.

Snapchat Strategy

Snapchat, now called Snap, is an app like Instagram. It is an extremely popular platform for the under-35 set. Actually, one of the big appeals of Snapchat to its fans is that, for the most part, their parents don't use it … yet. While users may skew younger, Snapchat users are growing up, and it has become a trend-setting platform for brands to experiment on.

Snapchat allows users to share pictures on their phone. You can control who gets to see and receive your images, and once someone receives your snap, it will be deleted after the timer runs out, which is set from 1 to 10 seconds only. The signature of Snapchat is disappearing content. Their claim to fame is the ability to send short videos, and to communicate through video chat. Their "My Story" feature allowed users to compile images or "snaps" into chronological storylines. This feature then morphed into "Live Stories" and earlier in 2017, Snapchat started allowing users to add links to snaps to direct viewers to websites.

Unlike Instagram, Snapchat users tend to be less interested in how pretty your snaps are and care more about the emotions and ideas they represent. The key is to be authentic, personal, and transparent. However, Snapchat does offer handy filters and editing features for novices to get comfortable with this unique platform.

Filters, including geo-filters that indicate the location of your snaps, are a huge aspect of Snapchat and allow users to customize and brand their posts. You can add colors, fonts, textures, animal snouts, flower crowns, 3D stickers, and even soundtracks, and more hacks pop up all the time.

Pros and Cons

For anyone over 35, Snapchat can be a cruel mistress. It is tricky to navigate from the get-go, and it is not abundantly clear at first glance how to use it. Mastering Snapchat can be challenging for impatient, distracted adults, especially with all the nuances, filters, and options that get added frequently. Becoming proficient using filters is a mandatory skillset to stand out on Snapchat. However, the platform is growing up and trying to appeal to a wider audience now.

If you are a private or introverted person by nature and tend to shy away from being in front of the camera, Snapchat may not be the best platform for you. Snapchat allows users to get an unfiltered look into people's lives, businesses, and unedited thoughts. Its raison d'être is as a powerful storytelling tool that offers a fresh way to send photos and videos to friends. In a nutshell, Snapchat involves snapping a photo or selfie, or a short up to 10 second video, drawing on it or adding text, incorporating one or many filters, throwing in some emojis for good measure, adding a self-destructing timer up to 10 seconds, and either sending it out to select friends or adding it to your Story. Stories is a curation of all of your snaps from the past 24 hours and then it is gone, unless you "save it down" in Snapchat speak.

Before you start snapping, chatting, or sharing your story, think through your mission and consider how Snap fits into your overall social media plan:

- Who is the prime audience you are trying to reach?
- What are their main interests?
- How can you engage your audience?
- What kinds of memorable content should you create?
- How can you use Snapchat to stay true to your brand?

Among the cons are the fact that Snapchat does not yet offer any real analytics to effectively track your progress.

Creating Stories

What users like most about Snapchat is creating their own stories. Stories are photos and videos that you can post to your feed that expire after 24 hours and can be replayed as many times as you want. Snaps, by contrast, are sent directly to select individuals.

Ironically, or perhaps predictably, Instagram unveiled its own version of Snapchat Stories that is nearly identical and rapidly surpassed Snapchat numbers in record time. So, the lingering question is now that Snapchat has morphed into Instagram, why do we need to be active on both?

To showcase your brand, create stories that feature:

Special Events: Preview an open house, share company or professional milestones, or promote a service or treatment.

Behind-the-Scenes Content: Give your clients a look at what you do for patients, share snaps of services you perform, share how you may select a skincare regime for patients, or give a tour of your clinic.

Q&As: Engage your customers and receive important feedback. Address frequently asked questions or pose a question that you want your audience to answer.

Sneak Peeks: Share exclusive content just for your followers, such as new, high-demand treatments, or post a snippet of a patient journey video as a series to illustrate what the outcome looked like on day 1, day 2, up until final healing.

Your Personal Story: Post photos and video snippets of a day in the life of an aesthetic clinic in order to give your audience an intimate understanding of what you do and the vibe in your clinic.

The following are other approaches to help grow your clinic:

Do an Account Takeover: Let an influential Snapchat user take over your account for a day. Consider asking an actual patient or colleague in a related field or a member of your clinic team.

Highlight New Blog or Website Content: Share teaser images and videos through a Snapchat Story, and let people know where they can find the full post or new feature. This allows Snapchat to act as a "trailer" for your website to spark interest.

Additional features on Snapchat include:

Memories: A cumulative archive of all of the snaps you have been sending and posting to your story and followers. Users can save their snaps on the app and share photos that were not taken "in the moment." You can create a searchable collection of saved snaps categorized by keywords, including location or an individual's name. There is also a password-protection section called "My Eyes Only," in which users can save more private/personal snaps for their friends to access.

Discover: This invites users to stumble on channels from a range of top publishers like CNN, Mashable, DailyMail, Cosmopolitan, Refinery29, People, and highlights current events and news stories in one place.

Things to Remember:

- Being on Snapchat can show that you are not a social dinosaur, but if your audience is not active on this social media platform, it may not be the best app to promote your business.
- The whole point of Snapchat is to be quick and in the moment.
- Snapchat is all about creativity and innovation.
- It is fine to skip a day or a few days if there is nothing to snap—less is more.
- Avoid starting lengthy conversations on Snapchat, because it does not keep a record unless you save the snap.

Snapchat Ads

Until recently, it was not easy to advertise on Snapchat unless you were a techie. It was not a user-friendly or speedy platform, because users had to reformat and convert their existing assets to fit into Snapchat's vertical video format.

Under pressure from Instagram, Snapchat launched a platform for users to create full-screen video ads quickly by using a web browser with a creative tool they call Snapchat Publisher. Brands can buy ads by using a self-serve buying option called Ad Manager.

This is how it works: Open the Snap Publisher tool, and click on the "Create a Snap" option. Choose your desired template, and upload your photos, videos, and logos to the templates, before saving and publishing your ads to Snapchat's Ad Manager. The Publisher tool allows advertisers to create Snap ads more efficiently by importing their existing brand assets and then being able to trim their horizontal videos to fit into Snap's vertical format. If they are so inclined, users can also select one scene to use for an ad.

Before you start advertising on Snapchat, build up a sufficient fan base who can view your content. If you are serious about Snapchat advertising, check out the new ad platform and choose one video to test so that you can see how long it takes to master. Then watch how it works for you, and judge whether the process is worth the time and effort. In my humble opinion, Snapchat is best managed by a millennial who really gets the platform.

We can expect to see more upgrades coming from Snap, as Instagram nips at their heels. As with Periscope and Meerkat that were hot once and died, these platforms are all moving so quickly that I think the better investment for clinics right now is Facebook Live.

Live-Streaming Video

The new flurry of live-streaming applications can bring your brand to life and bridge the digital divide between your practice and consumers. People are watching more and more streaming content. Live streaming refers to content delivered in real time, as events happen, online. It is akin to a live TV broadcast. To do this, you need a video camera and a microphone to capture the sound and images and a platform on which to broadcast the content. This can be accomplished with a smartphone or a tablet. With streaming video content, the user watches it live on a laptop over the Internet.

Viewers like to watch this evolving form of content for educational purposes, entertainment, or to learn about a product or specific topic. The challenge for busy practitioners is that this is a live event, as in right now, so it cannot be outsourced. Users demand authenticity, which means you will have to make time to schedule a Facebook Live session and be present to tape the video. Pre-video promotion needs to be done to round up viewers, although the video can be saved to view at a later time. Hold off on doing a Facebook Live video until you have a sufficient fan base to stream to, or you can use it as a hook and promote it with Facebook ads to build interest on your page. A typical Facebook Live session may last 15–20 minutes. If you are not getting people participating by asking questions on your page, you may end it sooner.

Facebook Live is the practitioner's platform of choice and has been picking up steam in medical aesthetic clinics. Since it can be done from an iPhone and is relatively straightforward, it is a good adjunct to a social media campaign and is growing in popularity.

To create a live stream on Facebook:

1. Go to facebook.com/live/create.
2. Click Create Live Stream.
3. Choose where you want your live stream to appear: your Timeline, a group, an event, a Page you manage, or a friend's Timeline. Click Next.
4. Copy and paste the server URL and/or stream key into the settings of your streaming software. A preview screen will appear.
5. Write a description, Video Title, and Video Game tag.
6. Click Go Live.

5 REASONS TO USE FACEBOOK LIVE FOR YOUR PRACTICE

1. Schedule a Facebook Live video session where you can answer questions directly to patients about a specific treatment
2. Give your fans a behind-the-scenes look at your practice, staff and a day in the life format
3. Generate excitement about an upcoming patient seminar or event
4. Introduce a new product, service, or procedure by explaining how it is performed and who is a good candidate
5. Broadcast biweekly or monthly videos for your fans about a variety of timely or seasonal topics—pull content ideas from your blog posts or create new themes

11

LinkedIn—The Most Trusted Network

The business of business is relationships; the business of life is human connection.
Robin S. Sharma

With sexier social networks sprouting up constantly, LinkedIn is a platform that often gets underutilized or put on the back burner. But it can be an extremely powerful tool if you take the time to uncover all of the platform's hidden features.

It is primarily focused on business-to-business relationships and enables users to connect and share content with other professionals, including colleagues, potential employers, business partners, and new employees. One of the best ways to be active on LinkedIn is to join groups that are relevant to who you are and what you do, such as aesthetic medicine and personal and professional interests, and to comment on discussions.

LinkedIn may not be as trendy as Instagram, or as popular as Facebook, but it is the most important social network out there for businesses. With over 500 million users and growing, if you are using social media for your business or professional growth, you cannot afford to ignore LinkedIn.

LinkedIn is technically *not* a social network. Its stated motto is "To connect the world's professionals to make them more productive and successful." It is not like Facebook; in fact, most serious LinkedIn users despise Facebook. It is a professional B2B (aka business-to-business) platform. That is, it was intended to provide content of interest to like-minded individuals of a professional nature. Perhaps more so than any other network, LinkedIn's purpose is clear. It is a place to connect with colleagues you already know and make new professional contacts.

They boast that one in every three professionals in the world is on LinkedIn. The operative word here is B2B as opposed to D2C (direct to consumer).

LinkedIn is not for reaching consumers. In fact, I would discourage clinics from using it purely as a patient marketing tactic. I often see search engine optimization people posting consumer blog content for doctors in groups on LinkedIn. Frankly, that is a good way to be disinvited from a group.

New LinkedIn Logistics

Microsoft recently acquired LinkedIn, which has boosted the networking muscle as the place where all business professionals hook up. The LinkedIn redesign is a far more sophisticated platform with user-friendly tools that help to reduce clutter and improve navigation.

In my opinion, the best way to use LinkedIn is to post in weekly updates about a workshop you attended, a great paper you read or research study you are involved in. LinkedIn is also a great way to hire staff and is ideal for job hunters. It is intended to help you connect with like-minded industry friends, colleagues, somebody you went to med school with, your community, and professional organizations.

LinkedIn Strategy

LinkedIn is really all about business, and I believe it should be managed by someone who represents your clinic internally or a marketing agency or PR firm. An important aspect of LinkedIn is staying on top of news and updates for brands that matter to you, and following influencers whose opinions you trust. Think of the vendors you work with, institutions you attended, and relevant organizations you belong to in aesthetics.

LinkedIn users are serious people. This is not a social site in the sense of the word. It is also not a community like Facebook, but it is great for disseminating and curating current information.

Since this is a professional network, the best times to post are during the workday. The hours between 8 AM and 6 PM tend to get the most traffic, and the best days are usually Tuesday, Wednesday, and Thursday. Posting on Monday can compete with start-of-the-week meetings and deadlines, so that may not be the ideal choice. LinkedIn's analytics provide an overview of the posts on your company page and a breakdown of your followers.

Creating a LinkedIn Profile

To get started on LinkedIn, create your "Profile" as an individual, not as a company. Your profile should be in your actual name—as in *John Smith, MD*, rather than *Smith Aesthetics of Surrey*. Just like with dating apps, adding a photo makes you far more likely to receive requests for connecting. To make your profile findable, start with a current professional headshot. A recent, professional, smiling photo of you is golden.

Include all of your current and past positions and education. These details will also increase your chances of getting found in searches. Listing your industry is also a vital piece of information. Complete your profile by adding any awards, research work, books you have written, studies being conducted, teaching positions, speaking engagements, preceptorships, and so on. You never know how people may connect with you, or what searches they may use to find you.

Write a compelling summary to explain what you do, and why someone should reach out to you. Leverage keywords by placing the best ones in key sections of your profile to improve how people can find you. Add at least 5–10 specific skills that speak to your expertise, such as plastic surgery, aesthetic medicine, cosmetic surgery, medical spas, clinical research, and so on. Last, add a brief summary of two to three lines that highlight the most important snippets you want your network to know about you. LinkedIn has automated feedback generated to help you build out your profile so you stand out.

To see how your profile appears to visitors, click on your photo on the top menu tab labeled "Me." "Endorsements" are also nice to add, and it is common practice to reciprocate.

By uploading a video to "SlideShare" and enabling it on your profile, you can also embed a video on your profile page.

PREMIUM PROFILE

If you are serious about growing your professional network, invest in a LinkedIn Premium profile. This upgrade allows you to see who is viewing your profile, gives access to advanced search filters, and offers InMail to reach out to people you may not already know personally.

6 KEY PROFILE SECTIONS

1. Headline—How you identify yourself
2. Current Work Experience—Responsibilities and activities described by keywords
3. Past Work Experience—Previous jobs or teaching appointments
4. Summary—Longer description of who you are and what you do
5. Specialties—Your complete skill set; Cosmetic Surgery, Laser Expert, Aesthetic Doctor
6. Profile Photo—Don't forget to upload a current professional headshot so your face will be recognizable to your network

Your Company Page

Establish your clinic or brand as a Company on LinkedIn. Go to "Work," and click on "Create a Company Page" to follow the instructions to set it up. This allows you to develop a valuable microsite for your brand, including employees, services, and content that extols the virtues of your clinic. You can select up to 20 specialties to highlight that are searchable—for example, Cosmetic Surgery, Aesthetic Medicine, Dermatology, and other relevant terms. Company pages can be used to post updates about industry news, speaking engagements, and clinic milestones to spread the word. This is a more appropriate place to recycle blog posts, media mentions, practice news, study results, events, and speaking engagements.

You can publish an original article or upload a link to an article you find online that is of interest to the users who follow you. Add your own commentary on the topic to personalize the content. Utilize share buttons to seamlessly post articles from sites and blogs.

If you are seeking a new aesthetician or practitioner for your clinic, post it on LinkedIn. To post a job, go to a Group you are a member of and post under Job. You can also click on Post a Job under the Work tab, and add it to your company page to get the best traction.

USING SLIDESHARE

Located under the Work tab on the top menu, SlideShare is a hidden gem. This platform allows you to upload slide decks about a specific topic you are passionate about. This is an excellent vehicle for promoting your unique expertise, for example, facial filler techniques, combination therapies for acne, using platelet rich plasma (PRP) with microneedling, or any other treatment or research you are interested in. The user can search by topics of interest to find your content.

Joining Groups

Joining groups that are relevant to you is a unique feature of LinkedIn to stay visible within your field. Go to "Work" on the top horizontal menu on the right, then click on Groups to search for new groups to join, and see what the groups you are a member of have to share. Most groups have open membership, and some will require you to request to become a member. Enter a term in the Search bar and click on "Groups"—such as Cosmetic Surgery—and you will see 156 groups for that category, 193 groups for Aesthetics, and 60 groups under Aesthetic Medicine. See which groups are worthwhile to join based on the scope and content posted. Groups are also formed around geographical areas, industries, companies, alumni groups, or any other social ties. If you are eager to build your local network, search for your city or country in the Groups search box. To connect with people in your industry, search for "dermatologists" or "aesthetic nurses," and so on. When you find relevant groups, join and sign up for the daily e-mail digest to get highlights of the group's activity e-mailed to you. If there is a question you want to answer, or help you can provide members, participate in the conversation. To gain from LinkedIn, you need to be present, and I don't believe it works unless you do it yourself.

Building Your Network

Many of your current contacts may already be on LinkedIn. Build your network by reaching out to people you know IRL (in real life).

Go to "Contacts" > "Add Connections." You can sync all your contacts from a Gmail, Hotmail, AOL, or Yahoo! account, which I do not recommend, or upload your contacts as a spreadsheet. Reach out to people already on LinkedIn, and invite them individually to connect. Personalize it, like, "I'd like to add you to my professional network on LinkedIn." By sending out individual invites, you can control the message by saying why you are reaching out and how you know the person, and start building your network.

Elevate your visibility by checking out the Answers section under "More" in the navigation bar. Search for questions from other professionals in your areas of expertise. Answering questions can increase your visibility and establish you as an expert in your field.

Applications allow you to add business presentations to your site or promote your business blog. You can also announce upcoming speaking engagements.

> **Keep your network confidential. Go to "Me" and click on "Settings and Privacy," go to "Privacy" and follow instructions to select the settings you want.**

LinkedIn Etiquette

The Right Way to Use LinkedIn

Content and stimulating conversations are the cornerstones of LinkedIn's model. In general, the best content encourages an open discussion, rather than just serving a thinly veiled vehicle for self-promotion.

How to Get Unfollowed on LinkedIn

As an early adopter on LinkedIn, it remains my preferred platform to spend time on and a key destination to stay on top of industry news and trends, and find out where colleagues are now working. I started in 2009, and my network is now 11,000 real colleagues and acquaintances.

Diehard LinkedIn users like me do not really want to see announcements about your new website, social events like birthdays, political statements, or a plastic surgeon being quoted in a local newspaper where they look for jobs, search for superstar employees, and hunt for new launches and interesting statistics or trend data. It is disrespectful, and diehard LinkedIn users will not be shy about calling you out on it.

If your social media or marketing agency is reposting blog content entitled: *5 Ways to Forestall Wrinkles* or *How to Get a Better Butt*, they are missing the point of what LinkedIn is all about. This strategy can backfire badly. Although it may be true that consumers also spend time on LinkedIn—after all, we are all consumers—this type of content should be discouraged from being shared on this platform. Use it on Facebook or Pinterest.

LinkedIn is considered a safe place.

12

Final Thoughts

Success seems to be connected with action. Successful people keep moving. They make mistakes, but they don't quit.

Conrad Hilton

Congratulations! If you have come this far, you have demonstrated a serious commitment to growing your clinic to be wildly successful. I sincerely hope you will face Monday morning with a renewed interest, ignited passion, and a genuine thirst to go further.

Following are a few final thoughts before I bid you adieu.

Technology was invented to serve people. The human touch is what drives technology. Don't forget that when you are feeling overwhelmed by your laptops, smartphones, tablets, and cameras.

Humans want to engage. They don't want to be talked at. They want to be heard. It does not matter whether it is online or offline.

Most practitioners do not have time to blog or tweet on a regular basis, so you may be faced with the choices of identifying someone on staff who can manage your clinic marketing, hiring someone to take it over, or farming some or all of it out to an experienced consultant. Although younger doctors tend to be more savvy about marketing and the Internet, hiring a full-time marketing director can free up physician time and increase efficiency. A marketing manager does all the behind-the-scenes work, so the practitioner can spend more time taking care of patients.

There are some aspects of practice marketing that still rest with the practitioner directly. You need to develop professional contacts in the community. Building a reputation and a solid referral base among your peers is paramount to success. Reaching out to other healthcare providers to create two-way referral relationships can be very helpful in building a practice, whether you are new or established. This is a social network that helps feed your practice and establish your reputation in the community.

Tech Medicine

Telemedicine is trending. This emerging field involves the use of electronic information and telecommunications technologies, including videoconferencing, e-mail, smartphones, the cloud, streaming media, and wireless communications. Using a desktop computer, laptop, tablet, smartphone, or landline, consumers are now able to get connected to healthcare providers from anywhere in the world without leaving their office or home.

However, in an age where e-mail exchanges with patients, electronic medical records, and cloud-based solutions are commonplace, the regulations governing these matters have a long way to go to keep up with how fast the practice of medicine is changing. This calls attention to how appropriate precautions that mitigate the risks of private information getting into the wrong hands must be taken, and to how physicians must learn to protect themselves. For example, third parties that are granted access to patient information may be required to sign a business associate agreement to ensure compliance. You will be wise not to take risks with your license or reputation, and make sure you are using the right technology to stay safe.

As technology continues to impact our daily lives, it will affect how patients get their facial injections, patients receive post-op care from facelifts and tummy tucks, prescriptions get filled, and skincare gets replenished. Walk-in, no-appointment-necessary clinics for Botox and fillers are popping up all over. Got acne and don't want to wait six weeks to see your dermatologist? No problem. A growing number of apps and websites, such as Klara and First Derm, are facilitating consultations by having patients submit a medical history questionnaire and a selfie to receive prescriptions from dermatologists within 24 hours for a nominal fee. Digital health is a fast growing field that is changing the way we live. Just look at the advances being made in genetic testing from companies like Arivale and 23andMe.

The consultation process is also undergoing a sea change. These can now take place in person, by phone, online, or through Skype, but none of these platforms are encrypted. More aesthetic practitioners are offering virtual consultations for patients who are traveling or have a tight schedule. Think of it this way—the more patients who are exposed to your practice, the more procedures will be booked. Patients are busy and less willing to travel far just for a consultation or to take time in their busy lives to spend time in waiting rooms seeing several physicians before making a decision. However, they may be willing to drive for a few hours or get on a plane to have a procedure with their physician of choice, based on his or her reputation.

What Does the Future Hold?

Telemedicine has the potential to enhance the patient experience. Patients can log onto a portal to view their records and request a prescription refill. Doctors can read notes from their office, their home, or while sitting on a beach somewhere. They can view x-rays and scans on a tablet or their Apple Watch, and do consultations and follow-ups on their phones.

It may take some time to work it all out, but we will get there eventually. Let's all enjoy the ride.

Appendix

Social Media Shorthand

In a world where 140 characters can cause an international incident, every character counts. One good way to don your social media clout is to talk the talk, especially if your target audience is under 35. If you are ready to take your social media interactions to the next level, these popular acronyms can help you communicate like a pro.

AMA: Ask me anything
Usually used for crowdsourced Q&A sessions.

BAE: Before anyone else
This typically refers to a person's significant other but could be a very close friend as well. It can also be used to denote keen interest in a product of any sort. For example, that lip filler is BAE.

BF: Boyfriend or best friend

BFF: Best friends forever
An oldie but goodie.

BTW: By the way

DM: Direct message
A DM is a messaging function on Twitter and Instagram that allows you to send a private message to another user. Tip: you can only send a DM to a Twitter or Instagram user who is already following you, and you can only receive messages from people you follow.

FBF: FlashBack Friday
A useful hashtag to use instead of #ThrowbackThursday (#TBT).

FF: Follow Friday
This trend began as a Twitter hashtag for recommending people who merit attention on social media. Most users save it for especially interesting shout-outs.

FOBI: Fear of being involved

FOMO: Fear of missing out
FOMO is the fear that you are missing out on a great experience, like a party, event, concert, trip, and so on. This is a cornerstone of the millennial mind-set.

FTW: For the win
Used to add excitement or emphasis at the end of a social post, but more often used sarcastically (e.g., "He missed his deadline again, FTW!").

FYI: For your information
Another classic that is still in frequent rotation.

ICYMI: In case you missed it
Catching you up on the latest information and news (e.g., "ICYMI, Beyonce had twins").

ICYWW: In case you were wondering

IMO/IMHO: In my opinion, In my honest/humble opinion
Especially popular in the era of "fake news" and fact checking, this is a way to clarify that you are offering your opinion, and that it is open to interpretation.

IRL: In real life
To let people know you are talking about something in the real world. Used to distinguish between the real world and the Internet world.

JK: Just kidding
Used to convey a light-hearted tone when there is a possibility for a statement to be misconstrued.

JW: Just wondering

LMK: Let me know
If someone writes this in a message to you, they are expecting a response. Also LYK—"I'll let you know."

LOL: Laughing out loud

MCM: Man crush Monday
A trend on social media where you reveal who your "man crush" is. It must be done on a Monday for the hashtag to have any meaning (and to optimize visibility).

NBD: No big deal
Aside from using it genuinely, you can also use it in a playfully facetious way (e.g., "I ran a marathon, NBD").

OH: Overheard
Generally used as a context for quotes.

OMG: Oh my God/Oh my gosh
Used to convey a bevy of emotions, most often surprise and excitement. Use the acronym where you would use the phrase in your day-to-day life.

OOTD: Outfit of the day
A popular Instagram hashtag, #OOTD means that you are showcasing an outfit you wore that day or an outfit that is suited for that day.

POTD: Photo of the day/Pic of the day
If you are in the habit of posting a daily photo on Instagram, this acronym is useful as a hashtag to make sure your photo gets seen by people looking for accounts to follow.

QOTD: Quotation of the day/Quote of the day
Theoretically similar to POTD and OOTD, a way to denote a post belonging to a series of daily posts including quotations.

Q or QQ: Question/Quick question

SO or S/O: Shout out
To credit/attribute something in a post, or to reference another person (e.g., "shout-out to my mom for raising me). It is like saying "kudos."

TBH: To be honest
When someone wants to emphasize that they are giving their honest opinion, often used for negative feedback (e.g., "TBH I don't like those sunglasses").

TBT: Throwback Thursday
A trend on social media where people post old photos of themselves or others on Thursdays (#ThrowbackThursday, #TBT).

TIL: Today I learned

More a hashtag than anything else, this is used to signal your post's belonging in a category of posts highlighting something you learned today.

TL; DR: Too long; didn't read

When someone has not read what you have written but wants to reply anyway. You can also use it to give a brief synopsis of a post or article.

TMI: Too much information

Typically used to respond to someone who has overshared (e.g., "Ew, Pamela, don't tell me about your UTI, that's TMI").

WCW: Woman crush Wednesday

A trend on social media where people reveal who their female crushes are on Wednesday. Like MCM, it should be done on the day stipulated by the hashtag for it to be relevant.

YOLO: You only live once

Another millennial mantra, YOLO is often said before (or after) you take a risk in life.

20 Ways to Bump Your Social Media Up a Notch

1. **Fill-in-the-Blank Posts:** Crowdsource to get a data point of interest (e.g., If I could have any aesthetic treatment, I would _____?).

2. **Behind-the-Scenes Photos:** Take candid shots of yourself or your employees, or snap a shot of your office or workspace.

3. **DidYouKnow Stats:** Share new, relevant statistics that are of general interest, such as "#DidYouKnow that 50% of women will start losing their hair before they turn 50?" Include a source or link for credit.

4. **Post a Link to an Old Blog Post:** Think about recycling good content. An older post can be reused to gain new engagement by extending its life and refreshing the content with a new hashtag or image.

5. **Quotagraphics:** Post a funny or inspirational quote and image branded with your clinic logo or URL on it. Include #QOTD (quote of the day) or #Wisewords.

6. **Infographics:** Find an infographic your followers would appreciate, and share it along with your comments, or create your own. Use a theme that will generate shares, such as "5 Ways Not to Hate Your Neck" or "Skincare Clinic: Key Ingredients Your Skin Needs."

7. **Product Photos:** These images perform best on Pinterest, Instagram, and Facebook. Add your own unique angle (e.g., staff member using the product, patient-submitted photo, doctor showing how to use it, etc.), and tag the brand.

8. **Recommend Your Favorite Products:** Share a list, photos, and benefits of your top sellers, highest-rated products, or the doctor's personal favorites to make it more personal.

9. **Offer Relevant Tips:** Post expert tips that your followers will find helpful. Add commonly used hashtags, such as #SkincareTip #FitTip #AcneTip #ProTip.

10. **Post a GIF or Meme:** Getting your customers to smile along with you is a good way to build your community. Search for GIFs or memes online by the action or emotion you want to convey, such as, an "eye roll," "I can't," and "here we go" or "RBF" (resting bitch face)

11. **Share Breaking Industry News:** Stay on top of what is going on in aesthetic medicine, dermatology, and cosmetic surgery, or offer a synopsis with your opinion on cutting-edge research as it arises.

12. **Share Your Predictions:** Consumers and media love predictions from experts. For instance, "The next big thing in medical aesthetics will be targeted fillers for lips and eyes."

13. **Profile the Staff:** Let your followers know something more personal about the staff they interact with. Give them a glimpse of the real people behind the scenes in your practice—from the bookkeeper to the receptionist.

14. **Share Photos from an Event:** Use the event hashtag for maximum exposure, such as #IMCAS2018, and tag any people (not patients without permission!) and locations in the photos.

15. **Create a Post Series:** Share a series of themed and numbered posts over a specified number of days, such as "10 Reasons Why Your Hair May Be Falling Out." This helps give fans a reason to come back for the next post on a topic of interest.

16. **Host a Giveaway:** Ask your fans or followers to comment on or answer a question or share their photo or experience to enter to win a special gift, such as samples of a new product, goody bag of products, or gift certificate.

17. **Offer a Sneak Peek:** Whet your fans' appetites by showing a sneak peek of an upcoming contest, new treatment, or product launch.

18. **Answer an FAQ:** Is there a question you get asked a lot by patients? Answer it on Facebook, create a short video for YouTube, or create a slide deck for SlideShare.

19. **Post an Excerpt from a Blog Post:** Rather than just posting a link and summary of the post, cut and paste a particularly intriguing excerpt to pique your readers' interest.

20. **Host a Video in Real Time**: Engage your fans by doing a Facebook Live video of a consultation or treatment from your Facebook page with a live Q&A period where you can answer fan questions. Promote the event throughout all social media channels.

Resources

These helpful resources will keep you up to date on new launches and changes to digital platforms and strategies:

- wendylewisco.com/blog (This is the author's business blog that is updated weekly.)
- Brainyquotes.com
- Businessinsider.com
- Emarketer.com
- Hubspot.com
- Huffingtonpost.com/topic/digital-marketing
- Jeffbullas.com
- Kevinmd.com
- Mashable.com
- Socialbakers.com
- Socialmediaexaminer.com
- Socialmediatoday.com
- Techcrunch.com

Index

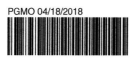